'Maggie La Tourelle leads us through a human and spiritual labyrinth in the language of the heart with her mother, who, though she has Alzheimer's, is at times intelligent, thoughtful, direct and wise. Her metaphors invoke the reader's deep involvement and the book provides a treasure of guidance to help us understand this frightening illness.'

Donna Eden, inspirational speaker, teacher and
pioneer in the field of energy medicine

'This book takes one to a deep level of understanding that could only come from personal observation. Maggie La Tourelle describes the gradual stripping away of personality by Alzheimer's, leaving the essential central core, as if one could see into the self and what is beyond. She gives a moving account of this dissolution process and the "thinning of the veil" that removes the barrier to another consciousness, and of the feeling that there are supportive though unknown presences always with you. A truly remarkable book that shows great insight and understanding and will be of inestimable help to anyone caring for someone with the disease.'

Peter Fenwick MB BChir FRCPsych,
consultant neuropsychiatrist

'Difficult as it may be to fathom, each of us plans a lifetime, including great challenges like Alzheimer's, before we are born. Why on earth would any soul choose to experience Alzheimer's or to lose someone to it? In *The Gift of Alzheimer's*, Maggie La Tourelle provides answers to that difficult question. Her poignant, heart-opening book is testament to the wisdom of what I believe is her and her family's courageous pre-birth plan.'

Robert Schwartz, between-lives regression hypnotist and
author of *Your Soul's Gift*

'*The Gift of Alzheimer's* is so much more than a book about dementia – it is poignant, profound and progressive in its ideas. It is a groundbreaking book that will teach you the language of people living with Alzheimer's and how to reach the person inside and bring out the best in them. As a teaching resource it is essential reading for all health-care professionals. This book will convince you of the need to connect to your emotional core and will open up the world of dementia like never before.'

David Sheard (Dr), CEO of Dementia Care Matters
and author for the Alzheimer's Society (UK)

'This moving and beautiful book will warm the heart and give insight to anyone interested in the mysteries of ageing and caring. Maggie La Tourelle provides an inspiring model of how to accompany someone through these crucial years in which deep and wonderful things are still happening, despite the apparent frailty of the mind and body. I warmly recommend it.'

William Bloom PhD, spiritual teacher and bestselling author of books including *The Endorphin Effect*

'An experienced therapist, Maggie was able to expertly interpret her mother's metaphorical and symbolic language, which allowed understanding and a meaningful way of communicating. Maggie's attention to these subtleties resulted in a great healing of their relationship for both of them. All too often such subtle cues go unnoticed because as a society we have been conditioned into ignoring them ... This is a very important book which shares deep wisdom and will be of great help and comfort to others looking after a loved one with Alzheimer's. It should also be essential reading for all healthcare workers.'

Dr Penny Sartori, author of *The Wisdom Of Near-Death Experiences*

'*The Gift of Alzheimer's* shines a hugely positive light on a condition popularly viewed as unremittingly bleak. Maggie's simple but profound advice ... will help anyone caring for someone with late-stage Alzheimer's, professionally or personally, toward a better understanding of, and a deeper connection with, the person behind the disease.'

The National Council for Palliative Care

'The love and humour used to manage situations arising through Alzheimer's demonstrate the ability to communicate in many different ways to reduce tensions and maintain the mother-and-daughter bond. [The book] provides the reader with many useful tips and advice on caring for a loved one with dementia.'

Dementia UK

'This book should be a necessary companion for any health and social-care student and warrants inclusion on any academic reading list.'

British Association of Social Workers

'A testament to the power of love in overcoming disease and dysfunction.'

Network Review, the journal of The Scientific and Medical Network

'This book makes a profound and original contribution to the field of dementia care. It is a story of the triumph of love over adversity.'
Dr Andrew Powell, Founding Chair of the Spirituality and Psychiatry Special Interest Group of the Royal College of Psychiatrists, UK

'Through a moving documentation of conversations with her mother, Maggie La Tourelle shows how attentive listening to someone suffering from Alzheimer's can yield profound spiritual insights.'
Linda Woodhead MBE DD, Professor in the Sociology of Religion at the University of Lancaster

'*The Gift of Alzheimer's* would be a useful reflection for any child of a parent diagnosed with dementia ... [La Tourelle] shows how to express the emotional responses to a parent's illness in an unconditional positive way. And when reading it makes you cry, remember that is also allowed.'
Royal College of Psychiatrists

'A brave and intimate book. Maggie has told her family story with compassion, sensitivity and respect ... Thank you, Maggie, for bringing this to the therapeutic world.'
The Psychotherapist, journal of the UK Council for Psychotherapy

'I fully endorse ... careful listening and understanding of people with dementia ... and for all those involved in Alzheimer's to be open-minded and more conscious of what is happening, aware of the wider possibilities, and know how to respond appropriately.'
Therapy Today, journal of the British Association for Counselling & Psychotherapy

'Like all good teachers, Maggie has the ability to make complex processes accessible to those of us who may not be quite as articulate ... using language that is simple, beautiful and honest.'
David Gordon Wilson PhD, President of the Scottish Association of Spiritual Healers

'An incredible and remarkable new book ... The words, emotions and feelings conveyed provide one of the most powerful insights into the world of a person with dementia.'
The Modern Registered Manager Journal

'A deeply touching and compassionate book that explores one of life's greatest challenges.'

Tim Freke, author of over thirty books
including *The Mystery Experience*

'Maggie was able to develop strategies to communicate, cope and find love in the experience. She provides ... advice that is being welcomed by leading doctors, charities and carers.'

Yoga Magazine

'*The Gift of Alzheimer's* offers an insight into a world so mysterious and final – it is compulsive reading. It is full of compassionate understanding and empathy and adds a surprising dimension, not only in Maggie's innate ability to understand what lies beyond, but in her ability to learn from it and explain this to others ... This moving, personal story offers the possibility for the sensitive souls of this world to go beyond the cursory hospital/care-home visit, to listen and learn and be truly amazed.'

Freda Robertson, a close relative
of someone who had Alzheimer's

ABOUT THE AUTHOR

Maggie La Tourelle is an eclectic and creative writer, therapist and teacher with a passion for life. She has worked in the field of holistic health care for thirty years, integrating psychotherapy, NLP, kinesiology and energetic healing. At a personal level she has ten years' hands-on experience helping to care for both her parents at the end of their lives.

She is the author of *Principles of Kinesiology*, which after twenty years continues to be a classic on the subject, and she has contributed to other books and international journals on holistic health care.

Maggie lives in London but remains close to her Scottish roots. Originally trained as an art teacher, she enjoys designing and making things, from greeting cards to clothes and furniture.

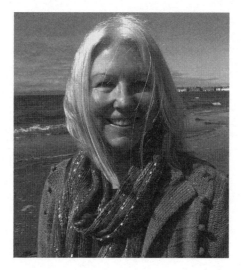

The Gift of
Alzheimer's

New Insights into
the Potential
of Alzheimer's
and its Care

Maggie La Tourelle

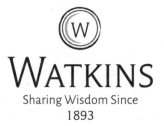

WATKINS

Sharing Wisdom Since
1893

This edition published in the UK and USA in 2015 by
Watkins, an imprint of Watkins Media Limited
19 Cecil Court
London WC2N 4HE

enquiries@watkinspublishing.co.uk

1 3 5 7 9 10 8 6 4 2

Designed and typeset by JCS Publishing Services Ltd

Printed and bound in Europe

A CIP record for this book is available from the British Library

ISBN: 978-1-78028-996-0

www.watkinspublishing.com

Publisher's note: The information in this book is not intended as
a substitute for professional medical advice and treatment. If you
are suffering from any medical conditions or health problems, it is
recommended that you consult a medical professional before following
any of the advice or practice suggested in this book. Watkins Media
Limited, or any other persons who have been involved in working
on this publication, cannot accept responsibility for any injuries or
damage incurred as a result of following the information, exercises or
therapeutic techniques contained in this book.

To my mother who gave me the gift of life,
and the gift of all gifts:
knowledge of life beyond.

ACKNOWLEDGEMENTS

I want to begin by thanking the various members of my family who have contributed, each in their own very special ways. My mother, the star of our story, whose need to know the truth, unconditional love for me, and deep wish to teach me, led me fearlessly on this journey into depths I had never imagined. Secondly, I want to thank my sister who, although not physically with us, was a key figure and without whom there would have been no story. And, thirdly, I want to thank my father who always welcomed me with open arms despite often taking a back seat during the intense periods when I was with my mother.

Cradling this story is the care home, and I want to thank all the staff from the bottom of my heart for the love they gave my mother and the support they gave me. I will always remember them with deep gratitude.

I want to thank Kathy Sorley for her editorial help in the early stages of the first edition. She helped me to discover the magic of words that breathed new life into my writing. I also want to thank Daniel Wallace for his editorial skills in the final stages of the first edition. He helped me to craft the book by bringing greater clarity to the organization of the material and to the content where it was needed. Finally, I want to thank my editor at Watkins Publishing, Fiona Robertson, for her superb editing. She added further clarity and made helpful suggestions that have enhanced the book greatly. Thanks also to my publisher Jo Lal and all the people at Watkins who have worked to bring this new edition into being.

My thanks also to friends and colleagues whose interest in my work helped to support me and whose suggestions were helpful: Gina Cowan, Anne Geraghty, Elizabeth St John, Ingrid Collins, Freda Robertson, Rosamund Irwin, Katharine Scott and John Sleeman.

CONTENTS

Foreword

You are holding in your hand a book that's perfectly wonderful if you know someone suffering from Alzheimer's disease – or if someone you know is dealing with such a person. If the second is true, you may want to pass this book to them the moment you finish reading it.

It is an extraordinarily challenging and deeply saddening experience to stand by and watch any beloved person encounter dementia and its particularly acute manifestation known as Alzheimer's.

In this remarkable book, Maggie LaTourelle offers her first-person account of such an experience with her mother. Yet this is more – much more – than simply a look at what she and her mother went through. It is a strikingly impactful chronicle that provides us with a window into the deepest aspects of this disease, how it may affect some patients and how it can actually become a spiritual gift to both the person afflicted and to family caregivers.

Frequently, the book's narrative surprises with totally unexpected insights and eye-opening glimpses into heretofore largely unexplored topics surrounding this disease – such as, for instance, what its deeper spiritual implications might be.

Its real-world, but oh-so-gentle, this-is-how-it-actually-is narrative places us right in the middle of the kinds of moments that others walking a loved one through these disheartening corridors are surely going to encounter (if they have not already done so).

The effect of this book is that of having a soft-spoken and truly caring personal consultant in the conditions of memory loss standing at your side in your hour of greatest need, providing observations and commentary that it is highly unlikely any staff member at a care facility will ever offer you as you deal with a loved one suffering dementia.

The most hopeful of these insights is what the author describes as her personal experience: that as in-the-moment memory capacity diminishes in some dementia patients, extrasensory and psychic or paranormal abilities can often be enhanced.

Alzheimer's patients very often present as being far more attuned to the emotions and energies of those around them than is assumed, and sometimes psychically 'intuit' what others in the room are going through, or are mentally absorbed by, without a word having been said about it.

The point that the author makes is that patients are very often far more 'present' than they may appear to be – and that knowing and understanding this can lead to more profoundly enriching moments between loved ones than might have been thought possible in these circumstances.

I can neither vouch for nor confirm the author's ideas here, but they certainly do open the Alzheimer's experience to a whole new level of possibility for patient, loving family and others.

As such, this book provides wonderful insights for those who may be feeling distraught or ill-equipped (or both) as they seek to meaningfully and lovingly engage with a person suffering acute memory loss and its accompanying functional disabilities.

Everyone who has had or is now going through this experience will thank Maggie La Tourelle for sharing this part of her life with such compassion, openness, understanding, generosity and love.

Neale Donald Walsch

Introduction

'We are all living in Other Worlds.'
Pat (my mum)

In the summer of 1997 I was walking along a beach on the west coast of Scotland, where my family lived, gazing out to sea with the wind blowing in my hair, when I was suddenly struck by the realization that in the next decade I would probably be facing the deaths of three of my closest family members: my sister, my mother and my father. This was a very bleak prospect, and I anticipated that I was going to have to cope with it on my own. I had a choice then to turn back and wait for it all to happen, or to continue on and prepare myself. And so began my journey of exploration into what many consider to be a taboo subject: death. I attended workshops and seminars, read books and contemplated this passage, one of the greatest of life's mysteries.

As a holistic therapist, I had an interest in all aspects of health and wellbeing and, living and working in London, had access to the information I sought. In 1999, my younger sister, who had been unwell for many years, died suddenly from an alcohol-related illness. A year later, my mother, aged eighty-five, was diagnosed with Alzheimer's disease, a condition that some would call a living death. By this time, both my parents were sorely in need of practical and emotional support and, being their only remaining daughter, I decided to make them my priority and support them to the end of their lives. I adjusted my life to accommodate these changed circumstances and so a new era began. I had no idea where it would lead me

1

and hardly dared to think about what might be looming on the not-too-distant horizon.

I am aware that the title of this book, *The Gift of Alzheimer's*, is a challenging and controversial one but my mother's Alzheimer's did turn out to be a wonderful gift to both her and me. Our story shows the potential there can be in late-stage Alzheimer's, and by sharing it I hope others can learn how to transform their experience of this devastating disease in similar ways.

Before we embark on this very personal journey, it is important to place my mother's and my experience within the wider context of Alzheimer's disease and dementia. There are said to be over a hundred types of dementia, of which Alzheimer's disease is one. It does, however, account for 60 to 80 per cent of all dementias and is the most feared. Like any family would be, we were very distressed when we received the news in the year 2000 that my mother had been diagnosed with Alzheimer's, for which there is as yet no cure.

Alzheimer's disease has been defined as having seven stages (see pages 228–30). Our Heart and Soul Journey starts when my mother was at Stage 6, moderately severe, and continues to Stage 7, severe, and to the end of her life. Alzheimer's is a neurodegenerative disorder causing damage to the brain that results in a plethora of neurological and physical disabilities, from forgetfulness, anxiety and an inability to manage complex life tasks in the earlier stages to rigidity, immobility and impaired or lost speech as the disease progresses. My mother experienced all these limitations and losses, but to our surprise and amazement she and I discovered that her Alzheimer's also provided us with a new opportunity, one we had not expected.

So what made this journey of discovery possible for us? As well as being my mother's caring daughter I am a holistic therapist, so I was able to bring my professional skills and expertise to the situation. My work addresses the whole person: the physical, emotional and energetic aspects. When doing psychological therapy, counselling and psychotherapy, I use a person-centred approach combined with Neuro-Linguistic Programming (NLP). I integrate this with a holistic system called kinesiology that uses muscle testing to communicate directly with the body and a range of healing treatments. I also do energy healing that works purely on the person's energy fields. I discovered that by employing these I was able to open up new channels in communication and wellbeing for my mother that had not been considered before or even thought to be possible. This may sound like the preserve of the professional but it isn't – anyone can help a loved one suffering from Alzheimer's and I provide information and simple guidelines on how to do this in the chapter 'A Positive Way Forward'. So this book offers a whole new way of approaching late-stage Alzheimer's. Through the mediums of dialogue between my mother and I, and my own commentary, it brings new understanding of the disease and will be helpful to all those involved with people who have Alzheimer's: family, friends, health-care professionals and educators.

Although this is a personal account of my mother and me as we faced her struggles with Alzheimer's and the end of her troubled life, it is also a multi-dimensional story spanning both this world and the Other World, between which she traversed seamlessly. As well as offering deep insights into Alzheimer's, this book also describes an exploration of the world of spirit and the life beyond that will be of deep interest to soul seekers and those curious about altered states of consciousness. It shows that Alzheimer's is a perfect vehicle for a journey of the soul and it is also a wonderful example of conscious dying.

The next chapter in this introductory part of the book, 'Event Horizon', provides the background to our story and sets the scene: the town, our family home and the care home that happened to be next door. It describes the events following my mother's Alzheimer's diagnosis: the physical and emotional difficulties, the real dangers, the inevitable denials, dealing with the authorities, and the impossible dilemmas we faced. Suddenly the *big move* took place and, through a blur of tears, I realized how final this was.

'Family Constellation' introduces the four family members who are part of our story: my mother, father, sister and me. It tells you about our characters, our passions and aspirations, our personal histories, our traumas and tragedies. My mother, the central character in the story, suffered from long-term mental instability and this impacted on all the family. Describing her struggles and passions brings me to explain my own healing transformational journey that started with the wounds I received in childhood and later led to my decision to become a psychotherapist and healer. My father, very popular in the outside world, faced irresolvable problems at home and was, for the most part, emotionally absent. My sister, damaged by early traumas, became an alcoholic and died prematurely, before the start of our journey. Despite this, mysteriously she turned out to be a key character, and without her this story would never have been told. Our histories also expose the constraining and unjust social mores of the time. All this information provides a potent backdrop for understanding what happens on our journey.

The central part of the book is 'The Heart and Soul Journey'. This is an edited transcript of the journal I kept and the audio recordings I made as I accompanied my mother during the last phase of her life, when she had late-stage Alzheimer's. When editing my journal, I aimed to retain the things she said and did that I thought were especially important and interesting, and to be faithful to the messages she was so determined to convey. Predictably, there was much repetition that I have omitted, but I have kept a few of her favourite sayings. Although, toward the end, our conversations were greatly reduced, I continued to record them as they provided an authentic and rare record of this end-of-life phase.

In addition to our dialogue, as my mother and I travel together, I interpret what she is saying and share my uncensored, innermost thoughts and feelings. So our story is intimate, deeply emotional and brutally honest, telling it as it is: the heartache and the ecstasy, the ups and the downs, the laughter and the tears. It shows that when love and compassion are present, the heart is touched and Alzheimer's can actually become a gift. At a practical level, our journey is also a vehicle for teaching how to deal with what arises with Alzheimer's. It is therefore not only very personal, but also universal in its meaning.

Remarkably, my mother retained her ability to speak, albeit sometimes in metaphorical language, and was able to tell me in her own words what she was experiencing, giving me valuable insights into Alzheimer's disease. But this is not only a story about our world. To my amazement, she experienced a spiritual awakening and entered an Other World. With an open mind, I listened eagerly to her as she led me boldly and unflinchingly, with a voice of absolute authority, on a boundless journey of the soul, teaching me stillness, mindfulness and other core spiritual lessons. Throughout, she gave me detailed information about the process of dying, life after death and the Other World. On many occasions she demonstrated exceptional extrasensory perception (ESP), and she regularly received messages from deceased relatives that enabled her to heal other family members including, ultimately, her husband.

One day, near the end of her life, she said to me, 'You talk to me. Nobody else talks to me.' Well, of course, other people 'talked' to her. She meant that nobody else talked to her in a way that was meaningful to her. In order to do this, I had to give her my full attention, connect to her with an open heart, and listen with an open mind. This is something everyone can do if they really want to, so I hope our story will demonstrate the importance of doing so and encourage others to do the same.

The final part of the book – 'Reflections, Revelations and Recommendations' – attempts to make sense of what happened during our Heart and Soul Journey and explores its implications for people with Alzheimer's, as well as the wider meanings from which we can all learn.

In 'Reflections on Our Journey', I acknowledge the particular set of circumstances that enabled so many wonderful things to happen. I look back on the lives of the members of my family and the dynamics that were operating before and throughout the final journey with my mother. This leads me to marvel at the deep healing that took place and appreciate that it was my mother's Alzheimer's and the transformational power of love that enabled this.

I also look beyond our personal journey to find out if what we experienced was exclusive to us or if others might be able to have similar experiences. My quest for scientific and spiritual understanding resulted in some interesting findings that I share in the chapter 'The Other World and the Neuroscience of Alzheimer's'. This research took me along a number of paths: one to recent research in the field of neuroscience, another to explore the laws of physics and another into the timeless realms of transcendence. I site my mother's story within a wider framework of altered states of consciousness, including near-death experiences, and other extraordinary end-of-life experiences, to show how transcendental states accessed in these circumstances offer insight into other dimensions of reality. So this chapter has relevance for all those interested in consciousness and the continuation of life after death, as well as people who are nearing the end of life and everyone involved with Alzheimer's.

The experiences of my mother and I, together with these findings, have important implications for everyone concerned with the care of Alzheimer's. In the chapter 'A Positive Way Forward: Care with Knowledge and Understanding', I offer a guide to looking after and being with someone with Alzheimer's. It contains a range of useful information drawn from medical and non-medical experts, Alzheimer's organizations and my own experience. I hope that this will be helpful to family, health-care professionals and educators, and that applying this knowledge and understanding will bring about the best possible outcome for everyone.

The final chapter, 'Closing Thoughts', takes a universal perspective, considering how the issues raised by this Heart and Soul Journey might be relevant to us all in our lives now.

EVENT HORIZON

'I have no past, present or future.'
Pat

Church spires dominate the skyline of this pleasant Scottish seaside town where our story takes place. Little has changed here over the years. As you walk along the beach and look out to sea, the island of Arran seems to float mysteriously just above the distant horizon. In the evenings, its majestic mountain peaks are silhouetted against the setting sun. People are courteous and nod politely, saying 'Good day' as they walk their dogs. On a windy day, kite-surfers add excitement to this respectable town as they race back and forth, sometimes taking off and flying through the air and performing other feats of daring. Sometimes horses can be seen galloping along the miles of sandy beach, and on a fair day the sails of yachts dot the ocean.

Summer visitors, many from Glasgow, flock to enjoy the clean beaches, the safe bathing, golf and the many little gift shops. Tearooms serve delicious homemade cakes, and the smell of fish and chips wafts from the harbour. This town was home to Dad's family and it is where my parents have been living during their later years. For me, this place holds many happy childhood memories: playing on the beach and in the sand dunes with my little sister and cousins. But this place called home, that sounds so idyllic, is also a safe haven for traditional values and attitudes that excludes those who rebel against them.

For years, my parents' lives continued more-or-less normally, until suddenly, overnight, everything changed. In 2000, following a visit to her local hospital, Mum was diagnosed with Alzheimer's disease. I was shocked by this news, having put her forgetfulness and slightly odd behaviour down to the distress of losing her daughter, my only sister, the year before. The next couple of years were very difficult. Mum struggled at home with

7

some additional help and attended a day centre. Dad, who was in his early nineties, and not the most patient man in the world, was battling daily with her challenging behaviour and was at his wits' end. I was living in London and visiting frequently, but things were changing all the time and it felt like a never-ending game of catch-up. I was often trying to manage arrangements from a distance, and needless to say felt constantly anxious and stressed.

Having successfully concealed her troubles throughout her life, Mum always managed to put on an impressive performance when the geriatric-care visitor made her fortnightly appearance. Sitting on the couch in the lounge, stroking the cat curled up on her lap, Mum would make polite conversation as if nothing was wrong – and of course to her nothing was wrong. Having been briefed by me about a catalogue of near disasters, our conscientious visitor would lean forward and tentatively ask, 'Do you want to go into a care home, Pat?' To which Mum would reply, 'No thank you', in an assured tone of voice that would defy anyone to dare question her further.

Behind this confident façade, however, Mum was not coping and, as her condition deteriorated, she started to pose a danger to herself and others. On more than one occasion, approaching our kitchen, I noticed a strange smell and discovered that the gas cooker had been turned on but had not been lit. Then Dad, whose sense of smell was not good, would come in and unwittingly go to light it, only to be stopped by me in the nick of time! Mum was outraged whenever we removed the tomato soup she kept putting lovingly in the cat's dish, unable to understand what she had done wrong. At night, she often refused to go to bed and in her nocturnal wandering occasionally fell and hurt herself.

I knew a disaster was just waiting to happen. When I informed the authorities of the risks Mum posed, they thought I was trying to push her into a care home prematurely and refused to take any action. They were carrying out their duty of protecting her rights, but for those of us who loved Mum and feared for her safety, as well as for our own, this seemed more bureaucratic than sensible.

Introduction

Our house happened to be situated next door to a privately owned care home. So, in February 2002, in a state of utter desperation, I booked Mum into it, ostensibly for a few days of respite care. However, I spoke to the matron in advance and requested that she carry out a full assessment. Within twenty-four hours, she called me back to report, 'There's absolutely no possibility of your mum returning home. I don't know how she's managed at home given her condition.' For a moment I felt guilty that maybe I had neglected Mum, then my feelings changed to relief. At last someone in authority had acknowledged the true state of Mum's health and the level of risk she posed. But in the midst of all this frantic activity, I did not prepare myself for the huge consequences of my action.

Mum didn't come home. Ever. Overnight she had become a permanent resident in the care home. Suddenly the house that had been her home and so full of activity, much of it fraught, fell silent and felt empty. 'What have I done?' Sitting alone on the edge of her bed, I could see through a blur of tears all the familiar things that said *this is Mum's room*. It was a sunny room, loved and lived in, with a general carefree untidiness. Taped to the walls were photos of cats and family gatherings, and drawings and paintings she had done. Labels with names and illustrations (which I had carefully put on everything to try to help her deal with her memory problems) adorned drawers and cupboards everywhere. Viewing all this, and knowing it would never be the same again, I felt utterly devastated.

As I took in the magnitude of what had happened, I wept. It was hard to imagine how Mum would cope with the strangeness of her new surroundings, the unfamiliar faces and routines, having been so confused and belligerent at home over the last couple of years. But to our amazement, she settled in well and was surprisingly compliant. I think on some deep level she was relieved that at last she was safe and was being properly and lovingly cared for around the clock. As is often the case with people in this situation, she had been in denial, fearful of change, and not knowing what she needed until she got it.

* * *

Having left the outside world behind, we now find ourselves immersed in a very different home, the care home, where the rest of our journey takes place. Buzzers constantly summon help, often more than one at a time. A heavy, sweet deodorizing scent pervades the corridors, masking more unpleasant smells. The noise of the industrial laundry machines can be heard running day and night. Wheelchairs are parked in orderly lines in the hall, and confused residents often struggle with the locked front door, wondering why they can't open it and go out. Some sit blindly staring into space while others, nearly immobilized, reach out to passers-by, hoping to engage with them. This is a place where people end their lives – a place where they come to die.

The care home is a large imposing house standing in well-maintained grounds, about a mile from the centre of the town. Its red sandstone façade bears the scars of over a century of prevailing wind and rain. Inside, its south-facing bay windows provide sunny panoramic views of the nearby golf course (my dad's second home), and beyond that, not far away, the sea. From its windows I can also look down, with some nostalgia, into the garden of our family home, just next door.

In the main part of the house, the rooms are large with high ceilings, ornate cornices and huge fireplaces, a reminder of the time when this was the private home of a wealthy shipping family. It is now home to thirty-two elderly residents and, like all such places, has its regular routines. Residents have breakfast in their rooms and slowly move up to the dining room for a very early lunch. In the afternoon, everyone sits in a circle in the large lounge, in varying degrees of consciousness. In the evening, residents remain in the lounge until bedtime, which for some, depending upon their frailty, starts immediately after tea.

Mum's room is in a new, purpose-built extension in the rear of this grand old house. When I visit her, if she is in the residents' lounge, I often take her to her own room where we can talk more intimately. Her room looks out across a patch of grass to another wing of the extension, but it is out of view of her old house so she could be anywhere. This is now her home and her world.

Introduction

The proprietor of this independent institution is a qualified nurse and sometimes works in the home himself. He said to me, 'I want to make this home a place where my own mum would be happy.' So, despite the overwhelming level of need, the staff members combine a high level of efficiency and professionalism with genuine loving care. Being long-term neighbours, my family and the staff know one another and enjoy a good relationship, one strengthened now that Mum is a resident. I am welcome to visit any time of the day or night.

Looking out of my bedroom window at the side of our house, I can see residents and staff moving around in the main hall of the care home just a stone's throw away. So it feels as if Mum is living in an extension to our house with access to all the professional care and facilities she needs, and I am reassured that she is in a safe, loving environment, out of harm's way. I can make frequent visits and spend lots of quality time with her. Dad and I no longer have to deal with her on-going unreasonable behaviour and he is able to regain a degree of order in his life. So, although traumatic at the time, we all quickly settle into this new arrangement.

With all these favourable circumstances, and my knowledge that when I am at home I am so close and on hand should there be any emergency, I feel very comforted. But this state of mind is shadowed by a profound underlying sadness about the long-standing tragedy of our family, the suffering we have endured throughout our lives, and the many difficulties that still remained unresolved.

In order to fully appreciate the gift of Mum's Alzheimer's, it is necessary for me to first introduce the family members who are going to be part of the journey, and to offer some insights into their lives.

FAMILY CONSTELLATION

'I love my family.'
Pat

This story, *The Gift of Alzheimer's*, comes to you as seen through my eyes. However, being a therapist, I am also bringing to it my professional knowledge and understanding. I have tried to be objective and to present fair, balanced and accurate accounts, but there is an inherent dichotomy in holding both these positions so, and at the end of the day, my account is subjective.

These are the family members, living and dead, affected by the journey I took with my mother, and by the painful struggles we experienced many years before this journey began.

Pat, My Mum

Although I know now that Mum started to suffer from depression almost immediately after I was born, I don't remember thinking that anything was especially wrong until I was about six or seven. I do recall that she was very anxious all the time. I couldn't understand why she found everything difficult, including simply leaving our house, or why she and Dad argued so much.

One day when I was seven years old, one of these rows spiralled out of control and Mum became utterly distraught. She ran into their bedroom screaming, 'I'm going to slit my wrists!', slammed the door and locked it. I was terrified as I knew there was a razor in the room. Standing trembling outside the door in the shadows of the dimly lit hall, I tried to speak to her but there was no reply. Time passed and still there was only silence. Was she lying dead on the floor in a pool of blood? My head was swimming, my heart was pounding and I could hardly breathe. I refused to leave her door, keeping vigil while Dad stood at the other end of the hall, rooted to the spot, clutching the phone. Eventually, after what seemed like a lifetime, the key turned in the lock and Mum emerged sobbing, unharmed, but with her spirit broken. This was the first of many such traumas.

Mum, Pat, was born in 1915 to a much respected Church of Scotland Presbyterian minister and a gregarious Irish mother (who, incidentally, was Protestant). Pat was the middle child of three: a son and two daughters. They lived in a thriving mill town in southwest Scotland. Mum confided in me that, despite Christian influences and a seemingly happy family, she had frequently witnessed tyrannical behaviour at home. Although in the context of liberal parenting today it sounds terrible, 'spare the rod and spoil the child' was the governing rule of fathers back then.

At school, she was a conscientious pupil who showed an early aptitude for music and gymnastics. She went on to study physical education, which she started teaching after graduation. During this time she met her husband-to-be, and my future dad, William. A dashing young army officer, William was drawn to this pretty young woman, slightly built, with beautiful wavy brown hair. They married in 1941, after a whirlwind courtship, the war allowing them little time to get to know each other. Apart from short periods of home leave, William was essentially away until 1946.

So, in 1943, I arrived in a fatherless home. After my birth, Mum experienced what she called a nervous breakdown. Today she would have been diagnosed with postnatal depression. She struggled on her own, not knowing if her husband would return from the war alive. Wanting to be able to stand on her own two feet as a married woman, she didn't seek medical help or confide in her family about her problems. However, she later told me that at that time she had feared she might compulsively push the pram with me in it into the nearby River Ayr. I know she loved me dearly, but her confession shows the depth of her depression.

Three years after my birth, and still suffering from depression, she gave birth to her second daughter, my sister Fiona. My father was now demobbed and home, so family life could finally begin. But it was not the happy existence to which she and Dad had looked forward throughout their years apart. He did not understand her depression; a former major in the army, he believed all she needed to do was 'pull herself together' and 'get on with it'. The tensions between them were never resolved, and my sister and I, caught in the middle, were inevitably affected.

The tyranny Mum had witnessed as a child, her untreated depression, being married to a man who did not understand her, and living in an uncompromising society: these all combined to destine her to a lifetime of depression and anxiety. Nor did she receive any treatment, as so little was known about mental illness in those days. Having lost faith in Christian benevolence as a child, she couldn't even turn to religion in her times of greatest need.

Throughout her life, although she appeared to cope on the surface, inside she was struggling and often very distressed. Her volatile nature led to spontaneous outbursts of uncontrollable anger during which she became a danger to herself and those around her. These were followed by feelings of despair, and on occasions she threatened to take her own life. Later, when she had a car, she would storm out of the house shouting that she was going to drive over a cliff and that we would never see her again. Hours would pass and we never knew if this time she had really done it.

When Mum was feeling well, she expressed her spontaneous, generous and loving nature, just like her Irish mother's, and our home was filled with music: singing, the piano and dancing. These joyful times gave glimpses of the woman that she could be, but they were never sustained. Her ego was fragile and the approval that she so desperately sought from her husband was not forthcoming. As a result, she felt inadequate and close to the edge, waiting for the next crisis to hit.

She made no secret of the fact that she found domesticity boring. But returning to teaching, which she had always found fulfilling, was not an option. Being the wife of a professional man meant she wasn't permitted to go out to work; it would have reflected badly on my dad's ability to provide for his family. She found the long-established, male-dominated social institutions intolerable. Having no way out only fuelled her anger and frustration and did nothing to ease her already strained marriage.

It was only when my sister and I were in our teens that Dad reluctantly agreed that Mum could return to teaching. Little did we know then that, hidden inside this anxious, troubled woman, dwelt a very different being: a creative extrovert and passionate dancer, like Isadora Duncan. And the timing of her return was perfect. A new creative dance movement, based on the work of Rudolf Laban, an innovator in contemporary dance, was being born in Scottish physical education. Fired with her passion for dance, Mum became a pioneer and one of the leading teachers in this field.

For years to come, she immersed herself in the subject, and it provided her with an outlet for her creativity and her musicality. She was a changed woman. Every spare moment was spent recording music and creating routines for children in primary and secondary schools. In addition to her teaching role, she was appointed to a pastoral position, guiding senior girls at the academy where she taught.

Sadly, during this time she also experienced a number of personal tragedies. First her brother committed suicide, having, like her, suffered from chronic depression. Then a few years later his son drowned. Following that, her sister, to whom she had been very close throughout her life, died of cancer. However, having found her inner strength, Mum endured these losses and carried on.

At the time of her retirement from teaching, a little granddaughter called Emily came into her life, the daughter of my sister, Fiona. Although the circumstances behind Emily's arrival were traumatic, Emily brought new happiness to my mum, and provided a much-needed focus for her love. My sister had become alcohol-dependent, and from the time Emily was born until just before Mum developed Alzheimer's, Mum was deeply involved in helping her daughter and granddaughter. Mum's need for companionship coupled with my sister's need for help and support resulted in a co-dependent relationship. Due to my sister's increasing inability to cope, at the age of eleven Emily was officially placed in the care of my parents.

In the year 2000, a year after my sister's premature death from an alcohol-related illness, Mum was diagnosed as having probable Alzheimer's disease by a consultant psychiatrist at her local hospital. The future looked bleak. She was aware that her body and brain were slowly disintegrating, and that Alzheimer's would eventually claim her life.

Me, Margaret, Maggie

I am Mum's daughter and her companion and faithful scribe on our Heart and Soul Journey.

Throughout my childhood, life at home was a roller-coaster ride: up and down and unpredictable. When Mum was well, love and joy flowed in abundance, but equally, when she was suffering from one of her breakdowns, her behaviour was often irrational and unreasonable. Her volatile nature meant she occupied all the family's emotional space – there was no room for me or anyone else. Determined not to be like her at all costs, I forced myself into an emotional straitjacket, and as a result refused to express any emotions openly at home.

Despite all these problems, I performed well at school and enjoyed a full, exuberant life outside our home. Yet, unknown to anyone as there was no one I could tell, following the death of a little cousin I started to suffer from crippling panic attacks. As I grew up, Mum and I followed the normal course of daughters and mothers challenging each other. But in our case that power struggle led to violent clashes, physical as well as verbal, which always ended with Mum in tears and me sorely shaken.

From a young age I escaped from the turmoil at home by losing myself in art and design. In my teens my focus moved to fashion and, although it had never been discussed, I assumed I would go to art school to study this. But when the time came, Dad, having experienced the terrible hardship of the Great Depression of the 1930s, refused point blank to let me go. He, like many fathers of his time, believed such places to be dangerous for their daughters – dens of iniquity. Furthermore, art school offered no prospects for job security. The options he offered me were to train as a nurse, or as a teacher or as a secretary. Dependent on him for financial support, my dreams were dashed. So by then I was not only doing battle with Mum, but with Dad, too.

Seeking a more exciting future than that planned for me by Dad, I joined a leading retailer as a management trainee. I made my interest in fashion design known and before long I was heading for a new orbit: London. And glittering it was, in the early sixties. Suddenly I found myself at the centre of the emerging fashion revolution. Reborn in my new life, I christened myself 'Maggie'. During this time, I was exposed to many new influences and one in particular had a profound and lasting effect on me. Friends introduced me to an esoteric group that practised transcendental meditation and studied Eastern philosophy. Each week we received material from a teacher in India that we discussed in our groups, prompting us to ask deep questions about the nature of reality. This enquiry and the new learning that emerged from it completely changed my perception of the world. Since that time spirituality has been the linchpin of my life.

However, despite my exciting new life, after a few years I experienced what I now believe was a spiritual crisis. The hidden wounds of my childhood started to bleed through their superficial dressings. Panic attacks returned once more, crippling me, and before I knew it I was tumbling faster and faster toward a black hole, with nothing to hold on to.

In those days, therapy was still the preserve of the privileged and little known in many parts of the country, but fortunately I was in the right place to find the intensive psychotherapy I needed. It took me on a journey into the dark night of the soul, where I gained deep insights into my unconscious. This process led me into Other Worlds where I discovered the rich meaning and revelations of dreams. The experience was profoundly healing and rewarding and I also found it fascinating. What started as a personal need, over time turned into a professional interest, sparking me to train as a counsellor and psychotherapist.

As I was emerging from my healing journey, I turned away from the razzmatazz of the fashion world and trained as an art teacher, returning to my roots as a maker of things. I spun and dyed wool, wove tapestries and rugs, and went on to become a studio potter. During this time, I met the man who was to become my husband. He valued and nurtured my creativity in a way that no one had ever done before. I was in seventh heaven. We had a son together and I embraced motherhood with every cell in my body.

Fulfilled with the joy of being a mother and my work as a craftswoman, I made a new and life-changing discovery. I found I was energetically sensitive. I was picking up on things in other people, feelings that I knew weren't mine; a phenomenon that healers describe. However, being a pragmatist, I was also sceptical. There was only one way to find out whether this intuition of my healing ability was correct – to try it out by attending experiential courses and workshops. So I embarked on a comprehensive healer-training programme, taught by a very gifted and experienced healer and psychic.

In one workshop on sensing auras, I discovered, when I held my hand in someone's aura and moved it through their energy field, that I could feel different sensations. This seemed to work as far as a metre from the body and as close as a centimetre away. I learned to interpret the different kinds of sensations I was feeling and how to balance a person's subtle energy to bring about a state of greater harmony. In another workshop, on reading auras, to my amazement I found that I could see the dynamic fields of energy that surround the physical body, and that these varied from person to person and from moment to moment. Through guided meditations, I experienced what seemed to me some very real past lives, something I hadn't believed in before. In another training session around this time, I had an extraordinary out-of-body experience, which I will never forget.

Having witnessed and experienced these various psychic phenomena, I was in no doubt as to the existence and healing

18

power of subtle energy and knew I wanted to apply this in my practice. But first I felt I needed some way to verify my intuition more objectively, for the benefit of both myself and my clients. This led me to studying kinesiology, a holistic therapy that uses muscle testing to assess all aspects of the person – structural, emotional, chemical and energetic – and select the treatment(s) that will bring these back into balance and harmony. My training in healing, counselling and kinesiology complete, I set up in practice as a holistic health-care practitioner, and later added integrative psychotherapy to my practice.

In time, my personal life changed, too. After many years, my husband and I recognized that we were heading in different directions, so we agreed to follow our own divergent paths.

Although based in London, throughout my adult life I visited my family in Scotland frequently, and when I noticed my parents' health starting to deteriorate I reset my navigation system to the north, to the sea, and to them. Although this might sound altruistic, I believe I was motivated by a deep need to try to put things right and heal the past. There was so much to heal.

William, My Dad

William, Mum's husband and my dad, was born in 1911. The elder of two boys, he grew up in a thriving town in southwest Scotland, where his father was a respected tailor. One day, when he was only eleven years old, he came home and on opening the door, found his father lying motionless on the floor, dead. I believe this shocking experience was imprinted on his psyche and affected him emotionally for the rest of his life.

William was a bright lad who after leaving school joined the Glasgow Stock Exchange. But the 1930s Depression halted his exciting career and he moved into the more secure world of banking. When war broke out he joined the army and rose to the rank of Major. During this time he met and married Mum. After the war he returned to civilian life and his career in banking.

Slim, quick-witted, charming, sociable and conscientious, William fitted well into the conservative society in which he lived and led an extremely ordered existence. He claimed his army days had been the best ones of his life; a time when he'd been out in the open, on the move and always facing new challenges. Back home, these needs were satisfied through his life-long passion, golf. He was a man's man and enjoyed the challenge of the game as well as the camaraderie of his fellow golfers, with whom he was very popular.

His second home, the golf course, was also the place to which he escaped when Mum was desperately crying out for attention. In a flash he would disappear, whack a few golf balls into the distance, then return home. This helped him to vent his frustrations safely. However, his repeated refusal to face his wife's emotional problems set up a pattern of poor communication that continued throughout their lives.

In this era, men and women had very clearly defined roles. If Mum had accepted her role, as most women did, her life might have been smoother. But being an independent-minded, creative individual, she rebelled against it. And it wasn't just differences of opinion about whether a married woman should stay at home or attempt a career that divided them. Like most men of his time, Dad didn't show his emotions, while Mum yearned for emotional connection. Feeling starved of love, she expected her husband to treat her generously in other ways but Dad didn't meet her demands. Having grown up in an era of austerity, Dad was cautious with money, while Mum spent or gave away every penny she ever had.

Even when it came to something they both loved, dancing, they were out of step. At the first beat of a traditional jazz band, Dad would be tapping his foot and clicking his fingers, while Mum, at the sound of ethereal music, would be floating around the room in ecstasy. And so it was, a classic case of 'Men are from Mars, Women are from Venus' – set in an uncompromising era.

To be fair to Dad, he found himself in a very difficult situation with respect to Mum's mental health. She was resistant to getting help and had he forced an assessment she might have been placed in an asylum, commonly referred to as 'the loony bin', where she would have been desperately unhappy. The stigma attached to this would have been incompatible with his job and position in the local community and he would not then have been able to provide for his family. But if he let Mum return to work, especially while their children were still young, people would presume he was financially hard up. And indeed, when, after many years, he reluctantly allowed her to go back to teaching, his best friend discreetly asked him if he needed some financial help.

In later years, being the epitome of respectability, Dad found my sister's alcoholism acutely embarrassing, and he couldn't escape from it as she lived in the same town. But when my sister was no longer able to look after her daughter, at the age of seventy-four he willingly took on the responsibility, alongside Mum, and provided his granddaughter with a secure and loving home. He tried valiantly to help my sister in his own way, though, sadly, to no avail.

Throughout our lives Dad and I had an unshakeable bond that grew out of our need, when I was young, to share our feelings of despair and anger about Mum. Although from time to time I strayed off the manicured narrow fairways of his course into the rough and wild of nature, in time he appreciated the value in my way of being in the world. As he got older he knew he could depend on me. His love for me, and mine for him, never faltered.

Following my sister Fiona's death, he never referred to her again. Maybe he had learned to cut off his emotions at the age of eleven, when his father died so suddenly. Maybe it was just the way Scottish men were in those days, having fought in the war for King and country.

Fiercely independent by nature, he continued to live in his own house well into his nineties. Despite the disabilities of old age, he soldiered on regardless, continuing to drive his car and playing golf nearly every day. But life has a strange way of teaching us the lessons we need to learn, and it made no exception for my dad.

Fiona, My Sister

Fiona entered our family constellation in 1946. She was my
parents' younger daughter, my little sister. As a small child,
Fiona looked angelic with her golden-blonde curly hair and
sparkling blue eyes. She had an innocence and fragility about
her that endeared her to everyone. At the age of two she suffered
a deep trauma. A serious kidney infection saw her whisked
away overnight to a distant hospital where she remained alone,
separated from her family and everything she knew, for three
weeks. Visiting was restricted to an hour once a week, in accord
with the barbaric rules of those days. I know now that it is
possible that this separation at such a young age contributed to
feelings of deep insecurity within her.

When she and I were children we were very close, and as
her big sister I tried to protect her from the troubles that were
continually erupting around us. I would take her away from the
scene and give her toys to play with in the hope of distracting her.
However, like me, she was exposed to our mother's unpredictable
and volatile behaviour and the on-going tensions between our
parents. There was no escape. At school, Fiona's performance
fell short of my father's high expectations and, being the second
child, she was not driven to perform like me. As a teenager I
continually pushed the boundaries and had endless battles with
my parents. Fiona, by contrast, was compliant.

After leaving school and a brief period working abroad as a
nanny, Fiona returned to the UK and joined Pan Am as a ground
hostess, looking the part in her glamorous blue uniform. In the
sixties, air travel was very exclusive and working in the airlines
was every young girl's dream. Through her work, she enjoyed
exotic travel and the good life, and it was in that world that she
met her first husband. But in her early twenties that same good
life led to her becoming alcohol-dependent.

After a beautiful wedding, she became pregnant. Her baby,
Emily, was born very prematurely and weighed only two pounds
at birth. A forceps delivery, relatively common in those days,
damaged Emily's tiny skull, causing slight spasticity on the right

side of her body. Emily is a survivor through and through, and no one would know she had suffered such challenges in her early life. Her mother, however, never seemed to find her own power and balance.

After a couple of years, Fiona's marriage broke up and she moved back home so that our mother could help with her baby. She married again, but this marriage also failed. Her drinking continued, and despite on-going support from everyone, and many abortive attempts to stop, she eventually lost the custody of her daughter.

Fiona's addiction to alcohol resulted in her life going steadily downhill. For a period of over twenty years I felt I had totally lost my dear little sister. Now we had nothing in common and nothing to talk about, and I found visiting her difficult. Her flat had a distinctive sour, acrid odour that I associated with alcohol, and the stale smell of cigarettes hung heavily in the air. On more than one occasion, when she opened the cupboard to get some tea bags, I could see there was only the minimum of food.

Aware that I didn't approve of her drinking, when she knew I was coming up to visit, she would suddenly stop drinking, going one hundred per cent cold turkey, and on two occasions I found her lying on the floor due to sudden total alcohol withdrawal. I felt guilty, as I knew I had inadvertently caused these blackouts. Following those incidents, whenever I went to visit her, my heart would pound as I stood outside her door, wondering what I might find on the other side.

Everyone tried to help Fiona. Being generous by nature, Mum gave her money for food – those well-meaning funds only serving to exacerbate her drinking problem. I tried to talk to her but to no avail. Dad paid for her to have treatment and Social Services worked tirelessly with her for many years. But alcohol addiction is a cruel disease – it takes over the lives of its victims. Fiona was no exception and over time she spiralled down and down into the abyss.

One day when I was abroad, I received an urgent phone call telling me that Fiona was in intensive care. Unknown to me, she had been admitted to hospital two days before, suffering from acute pancreatitis, an alcohol-related illness. I dropped everything, bundled myself into a taxi and got the next flight home. I knew Fiona didn't have the reserves to survive long and feared I would soon be dealing with the first of the family deaths I had anticipated.

Standing outside the locked doors of the intensive care unit, my heart felt as if it was going to jump out of my body. Sudden flashbacks reminded me of the times I had stood outside Fiona's front door, fearing what I might find, and also as a child when I had waited outside my parents' bedroom door, wondering if my mother was dead on the other side. Here I was again.

My parents were too old and too frail to deal with their daughter's imminent death, and Emily was unprepared and in shock. But I had learned at an early age to cope, and now I had to muster all my inner resources. Two days later, I gave the doctors permission to switch off my sister's life-support machine. Fiona died, aged fifty-three, with me by her side.

Six months before Fiona's death, she had proudly presented Mum with a carefully chosen Christmas present. It was a large framed picture of an angelic-looking young woman with a sad and fragile demeanour, dressed in a long flowing gown, suspended just above the ground with outstretched arms. Superimposed on this ethereal figure was a pattern that looked like the black outlines of crazy paving.

This disturbing picture, with its poignant imagery, encapsulated the tragedy of Fiona's life and is etched on my psyche to this day. Despite the numbing and dumbing effects of alcohol, Fiona knew her fate with absolute clarity, albeit at an unconscious level, as she approached her death. Although none of us recognized this at the time, it is now crystal clear to me that Fiona's gift to her mum was actually an announcement of her impending death.

Years later, in the care home, Mum told me something utterly unexpected and astonishing about Fiona. She revealed what might have been the true purpose of Fiona's life, without which our story, with all its mysteries, would never have been told. As you travel on our Heart and Soul Journey, you, too, will discover what this purpose is.

Breaking the Rules

It is not customary for us canny Scots, particularly of my parents' generation, to expose our personal lives in the way I am doing in this book. My justification for 'breaking the rules' is to fulfil my mother's expressed wish that others might learn from our experiences. In order for the profound healings that occurred to be fully appreciated, I have had to tell the personal stories of my family members and explain the dynamics that were operating. It is with some reluctance that I have written so honestly about my family and myself. The names of some of the people have been changed to protect their identity.

Venturing Forth

With all these thoughts in mind, as we travel lightly, perhaps tentatively, if we look, listen and feel, we will discover things that might seem impossible. So I invite you now to step out of the ordinary into the extraordinary, and, with an open heart and an open mind, join my mother and me on our boundless Heart and Soul Journey.

The Heart and
Soul Journey

INTRODUCTION TO OUR JOURNEY

'A rush of illuminations, lots of light.'

Pat

2003

It is summer and I am visiting Mum in the care home. She has been here for nearly a year now, and I am noticing each time I visit her how increasingly frail she is.

Seeing her in this weakened state, I am reminded of a critical event that happened nine months ago. I was asleep in my flat in London when I was awakened at 3am by my phone ringing. It was the night sister at the care home. She told me that on their half-hourly rounds the staff had found Mum deeply unconscious, and after many attempts had still failed to revive her. A doctor had been called and someone would let me know as soon as they had any news. An hour later my phone rang. My heart pounding, I listened anxiously to the doctor. She told me that Mum had come round and, to everyone's complete amazement, did not appear to have suffered any ill effects. She explained that Mum had probably suffered a transient ischaemic attack (TIA), a mini-stroke, common in people of her age, and that more could follow.

Recalling this event, which took Mum so near to death last November, I am aware of her vulnerability, and of the need for me to be more attentive. I decide, therefore, to cancel an upcoming holiday abroad so that I can be with her. As I am staying next door, I can pop into the care home frequently and spend lots of time with her. Fortunately, she picks up and is well enough for me to take her out in the wheelchair for walks and to bring her round to the garden of our house. As a result of all this contact, I am feeling a lovely closeness beginning to develop between us.

(*Note*: As you read our conversations you may notice that sometimes our dialogue doesn't flow in the way a normal conversation would. This is because of my editing. However, I have sacrificed nothing of the heart of the content and the journal entries are exactly as I recorded them, warts and all.)

OUR JOURNEY BEGINS

'It's difficult working between two worlds.'
Pat

Saturday 16 August 2003

I find Mum sitting comfortably in a chair in her room. She has
a bed, two chairs, a wardrobe, a chest of drawers and a bedside
table, all standard fittings. But the room is warm and cosy, with
many reminders of the past. Photos of family and friends have
migrated to these walls. A colourful patchwork blanket, knitted
by Mum for me, now hangs on the back of her chair. On top
of the chest of drawers sits an open box of ginger chocolates,
Mum's favourites, along with miscellaneous fragrant toiletries
and a collection of greetings cards bearing messages of love.

Despite everything, Mum looks good for someone of eighty-
eight years. Her searching blue eyes strike you first, vivid
against her colourless skin and her white, short hair. She has
the characteristic slight build of someone who has suffered a
lifetime of anxiety and, although the ravages of Alzheimer's have
rendered her weak and more or less wheelchair-bound, she holds
herself well, with an air of gentle graciousness.

Today, she is dressed in a blue cardigan that makes her eyes
look even more vivid than normal. A pleated skirt hangs loosely
around her spindle-thin legs, making her feet, nestled in soft fawn
slippers, appear disproportionately large. Her hair is nicely done,
having just been washed and set by the visiting hairdresser.

As I enter she smiles, obviously pleased to see me. I give her
a kiss and pull a chair close to her so I can look into her face and
hold her delicate hand.

Me: *Hello Mum. It's lovely to see you. How are you? How are
you feeling?*

Mum: *Fair.*
You love me, Margaret.

I feel touched by her very direct remark – she is saying exactly what she is thinking. She is so frail now and I am feeling deep compassion for her. It is not clear if her comment is a statement or a question, or both. Whatever it is, I know I need to reinforce her positive observation.

(*Note*: Although I have long called myself Maggie, my parents have always called me Margaret, the traditional Scottish name that is my given name.)

Me: *Yes Mum, I do.*
Mum: *I've always done my best.*
Me: *Yes, I know you have.*
Mum: *I'm a bad person.*
Me: *Oh Mum, how can you say that? You're lovely. You're a good person.*

This has come completely out of the blue and I feel sad that she is feeling like this inside. Why today? Why now? I wonder what the trigger has been. She is so vulnerable and struggling gracefully, without a word of complaint, to cope with a devastating and irreversible disease. There is nothing bad about her. My heart goes out to her and I want to reassure her and put it all right. But, as she and I had such troubled times in the past, I have a strong suspicion as to where this thought might have come from. Was it triggered by my arrival? This idea is causing me to feel slightly challenged.

As a result of Alzheimer's, it seems that the veil that separates her conscious and unconscious mind is thinning, allowing old thoughts from her unconscious to surface. Responding to what seems like an invitation to open a conversation, I find myself in the unusual position of relating to her as her daughter and, at the same time, as a therapist. I tell her that we can talk about anything she wants and she welcomes this, showing the trust she is placing in me. I am acutely aware of the responsibility that this brings.

Leaning forward in her chair, her eyes searching my face, she nods, agreeing, and looks eager for me to continue. We range over many different topics, including our relationship. Holding her hand, I tell her I know she suffered terribly from nerves and that made life very difficult for her ... and for all of us. I go on to tell her that she would have done things differently if she could have done. It's easy to look back now and wish life had been different, but she did the best she could at that time. Revisiting the past without judgement enables her to face the things that have been troubling her: her violent uncontrollable outbursts, her threatened suicides. To my amazement, in one conversation we cover ground that would normally take months in therapy.

The experience is emotional and at the same time affirming and healing for both of us. I am so pleased she is open to this honest exploration and I actually look forward to more frank discussions like this in the future. I never anticipated that we would have this chance to bare our souls with one another, let alone the inclination.

Following our 'therapy' and reconciliation, Mum honours me by saying:

Mum: *You have wisdom, Margaret.* [With a voice of real authority] *You have lots of time to do good.*

What a wonderful parting message! How does she know this? I float back to our house and drift up to bed, uplifted by this newly found connection with Mum, marvelling that it is happening in the shadow of her Alzheimer's. I am struck by the change in Mum and by the things she is saying. They are heart-warming and a little unusual so I decide to note them down. This marks the beginning of my journal.

With the reassurance of these positive experiences with Mum, I leave for London, looking forward to returning in a few weeks.

(*Note*: The dates of my journal entries denote when I am with Mum, while a line below each section indicates when I have been away and come back. During these absences I try to speak to her on the phone every day. When I return from my busy life in London it takes me a little time to slow down and 'tune in' to her again. Also it is likely, as she has Alzheimer's, that changes will have occurred during these intervals.)

Saturday 6 September 2003

It is evening and I have just arrived from London. I am visiting Mum, who is sitting up in bed.

Me: *Hello Mum. It's lovely to see you. How are you? How are you feeling?*

I am reciting a similar greeting each visit, so as to establish familiarity and a comfort zone for Mum.

Mum: *Average, Margaret.*
       You have a lovely face. Your blonde hair is lovely. Your teeth are lovely. Look after them – you only have them once.
Me: *Thank you, Mum, I will.*

I appreciate her compliments as they come out of genuine affection. Because she has Alzheimer's, she is commenting on what she is seeing without the normal filtering or censoring that we employ before speaking. It feels strange to have someone talk about me so directly.

Mum: *I feel so idle. I know I should be doing something. It doesn't feel right having nothing to do. What should I be doing, Margaret? Who is looking after the house?*

34

Me: *Don't worry Mum, everything is being taken care of. You've worked hard all your life and it's time for you to relax now and enjoy having no responsibilities.*

This is a recurring anxiety of Mum's but after we have talked about it she relaxes and moves on to:

Mum: *I often dream. My dreams are friendly, clear ... free, make-believe, bliss.*
Me: *Tell me about them.*
Mum: *I learned things in my childhood that help me now.*
Me: *What things, Mum?*

She can't tell me but then goes on:

Mum: *When you see little bits floating, flying off, you will know it's me.*

I am trying to imagine this. I think she may be seeing herself in energy form when she is no longer here physically. Might she be referring to energy orbs, specks of light that appear momentarily, seemingly from nowhere, and disappear again? How mystical!

I am stroking her. Being an energy therapist, and having understood Mum's remark about 'little bits flying off' to be a description of her energy, I immediately tune in to her aura, the invisible energy field that surrounds her body. I connect to Mum's aura with my mind.

Mum: *You are so good. You have a lovely touch.*
Me: *Something more is happening.*
Mum: *What do you mean?*
Me: *Our energies are connecting, lovely connections, Mum. It's good!*
Mum: [Closes her eyes] *Yes, that's wonderful.*
I'm not dead. It takes time. I'm not ready yet.

35

She senses this connection and likes it. This is the first time she has mentioned dying explicitly and I am a little shocked, although greatly relieved to hear she is not going yet. Her comment about death suggests I had guessed correctly – she was thinking about herself in energy form after she has died.

Mum: *I want to dance.*

Mum loves the composer Debussy so I am playing a CD of *Clair de Lune* for her. The floaty, other-worldly music expresses everything that she is as a dancer. In the past, on hearing this music, she would have spontaneously got up and danced unselfconsciously around the room, much to the embarrassment of my dad, who would have buried himself in his newspaper until the end of her gleeful display.

Me: *Shall I help you to get up and dance, Mum?*
Mum: *I don't need any help.*

Earlier in the day, Mum said she didn't need a wheelchair, although in reality she very much did. This refusal of assistance suggests she is perceiving herself as she was, rather than as she is now.

Mum: [Emphatically] *Dreams – the truth. They must tell the truth!*
       I don't want to do anything wrong.

Throughout her life, Mum has been a person of real integrity and someone who always sought the truth. So, true to character, she is seeking the truth now and doesn't want to do anything wrong. This seems to be a time for putting things right.

Not all dreams have great significance but most of us have at some time had a special dream that conveyed an important message.

Mum and I are having a lot of prolonged eye contact. I have noticed that she often fixates on things and I imagine this is due to her brain activity slowing down.

Me: [Breaking our silent connection] *Thank you for teaching me.*
Mum: *What?*
Me: *About being in the moment.*

When Mum stares at me with her unfaltering gaze, I enter a state of stillness, of being in the moment and totally present. I am in a timeless zone, a sacred space. I learned about such altered states of consciousness many years ago and little did I know then that I would be sharing this experience with her now.

Me: *You're a free spirit and will always be.*

I am remembering Mum's pioneering spirit and her struggle to express herself in a very constrained society. She mentioned the word 'free' earlier in the conversation and I want to help her to connect to her spirit and know that it is still free even if her body is not.

My own spiritual journey is contributing to my understanding of what Mum is saying and what is happening to her, as well as prompting many of my responses, questions and comments.

Me: *What is the lesson I need to learn?*

I am acknowledging that she, too, has wisdom.

Mum: *Being true in the moment.*

What a profound reply! There is a lot of silent eye contact during this time and we can look at each other without anything coming between us. It is very pure and feels like the moment of truth that she is telling me about.

Tuesday 23 September 2003

I have been away in London and have just returned. It is evening and Mum is in her room. She looks eager to talk.

Me: *Hello Mum! It's lovely to see you. How are you? How are you feeling?*

Mum: *Fine, thank you, Margaret.*

You may have noticed that Mum's response to my familiar opening greeting is either 'fair' (meaning 'not so good'), 'average' (meaning 'OK') or 'fine' (meaning 'very good'). Mum seems to be drawing here on the terms she would have used in the past as a teacher assessing her pupils' work. Her response is helpful to me as it gives me an instant reading of how she is feeling and enables me to respond to her appropriately.

My greeting has also become a prompt for her to start telling me what is on her mind.

Mum: *It's difficult being ... working between two worlds.*

Me: *Two worlds – tell me more, Mum. I'm really interested.*

No reply.

Is this a hallucination, a delusion or a profound connection to another dimension? Mum's statement comes as a complete bombshell. I can't wait to hear more. It seems that she is presenting me with an important choice: either to stay firmly fixed in this world or to be open to her experience of another world and explore this with her. If I opt for the latter, I realize it will set a precedent for the rest of our journey.

I notice that she said '*being*', then corrected this to '*working* between two worlds'. So she knows she has work to do. I am curious as to what this might be and wonder what other mysterious pronouncements will come forth.

Mum: *I have patience.*
Me: *Yes, that's true Mum, you have.*

I'm glad to hear her talking in such an affirmative manner about herself, especially after her self-deprecating remarks just a month ago.

I reflect on how far we have come together during the last few weeks. Our journey started when Mum wasn't well and she and I began to grow closer. She faced some old emotional traumas and we found reconciliation. Then we connected with the subtle energy dimensions – and that seemed to extend her consciousness to another world! Now she is proclaiming that she has the virtue of patience.

She certainly is finding her own voice and I am delighted to be witness to and part of this empowering process, especially as Alzheimer's disease so often strips a person of power, eventually reducing him or her to silence and a state of seeming nothingness. I am beginning to wonder if, instead, Mum might be experiencing a process of evolving into another state of consciousness.

Having left Mum in the care home, I walk up the path to our house thinking that I must tell Dad about Mum's amazing announcement about two worlds. At ninety-two and nearing the end of his life, he, too, should be thinking about these things.

I enter the living room and Dad is leaning forward in his chair, eyes glued to the television, watching a very exciting golf match. Pleased to have my company he starts giving me a running commentary on every stroke. Suddenly, I am very much in this world, his world. Where is the Other World now? It seems far, far away. When the match has finished I think again about Mum's pronouncement and wonder how I might open a conversation with Dad about the Other World.

But something holds me back. That channel seems completely switched off, not available.

EXTRAORDINARY HEALING
TREATMENTS

'I have access to a, like a first-aid box. I can go to it
at any time and get whatever I need.'

Pat

Wednesday 24 September 2003

Evening. Mum is in bed looking very comfortable, drifting in and
out of sleep. I sit down beside her and hold her hand.

Me: *Hello Mum. It's lovely to see you. How are you? How are*
      you feeling?
Mum: *Fine.*
      It's difficult. I've had a big operation. They have taken
      things out.

This is a curious announcement. Has she just had a dream? The
experience has seemingly happened overnight and could be the
effect of the emotional clearing she and I are doing together, but
she refers to 'they', suggesting the involvement of more than one
person and not including me. Given her previous statement about
working between two worlds, I am taking a leap and wondering
if the source is her Other World.

Me: *Where have they taken things out, Mum?*
Mum: *My mind. They are very skilful.*

As I thought, this operation was not pathological.

Me: *Who are they?*
No reply.

Might 'they' be *helpers* from the Other World?

Mum: [Emphatically] *Freedom is important, and patience.*

I am keeping a note of all the things that Mum is telling me are important.

Since our honest exchange last month about our past difficulties and the reconciliation that followed, I am noticing that Mum is being more open with me. Her language has changed, too. It seems that we are now on a philosophical and spiritual journey together.

Mum: *I'll soon be better. I don't like not being able to move around.*

In the physical world, poor Mum is very disabled now and more or less wheelchair-bound. As a former dancer and physical education teacher, these physical limitations are particularly difficult for her, I imagine. I wonder whether she is seeing herself getting better in this life or in her Other World.

After my visit I go straight home, review my notes and the tape recording while everything is still fresh in my mind, and write them up in my journal. I am doing this after every visit. Writing up the notes of a therapy session is something I do routinely in my work as a psychotherapist, so it is a familiar practice for me. It also gives me time for reflection and the opportunity to consider the possible deeper meaning of what Mum is saying and what is happening between us.

Saturday 18 October 2003

I am back in Scotland again. Mum is suffering from another urinary tract infection (these are very common in people with Alzheimer's). She is in her room, sitting up in bed and looking weak and frail.

41

Me: *Hello Mum. It's lovely to see you. How are you? How are you feeling?*

Mum: *Fair, Margaret.*
      My visitors, two women, they talk to me. They come about twice a week.

Me: *Who are they? What do they say? Do they reassure you?*

Mum: [Emphatically] *I don't need reassurance!*

The certainty with which she says this is reassuring to me.

I wasn't aware of her having two regular female visitors, so I check by asking a member of staff about her statement. They tell me that she hasn't had any such visitors. So who are these two who come regularly and talk to her?

Mum looks poorly and in need of rest. I need to have patience and trust that more will be revealed to me in time.

Sunday 19 October 2003

Evening. Mum is in bed and she is looking much more alert than yesterday. I give her a bunch of lilies and their beautiful fragrance fills her room. She appreciates flowers so I always make sure she has fresh ones when I am here, and I leave a flowering plant in her room before I leave for London. I am stroking her brow.

Mum: *So soothing. That's the thinking part of my brain.*

She is correct. I wonder if she has intuited this connection through my touch.

Mum: *You have a beautiful face. Your teeth are so white. Look after them. You are strong, steady, steady. Your eyes don't blink. You have piercing eyes. You have a strong body. That's a lovely jumper.*

Me: *Thank you, Mum. You are lovely, too.*

Mum: *You are such a comfort, such a companion Margaret. You are good.*
      She repeats this many times.

Me: *I love spending time with you, Mum.*

This is absolutely true – she is a joy to be with. I love her spontaneity and directness and I am very curious about the mysterious things she is telling me.

Mum: *This is a lovely way to say goodbye.*

I kiss her and I cry. I don't want her to go.

Mum: *Cry as much as you like.*
Me: *Tears of love, Mum.*
Mum: *I'm ready to leave – in a few days. Is that all right?*
Me: *Yes.*

My 'yes' is a very feeble one. Of course I don't want her to leave yet but I don't want to hold her back if she is ready. I know people who are ready to die sometimes hang on because someone close to them is not ready to let go.

Mum: *I'll sleep away. Don't cry for me.*
     I have relatives visit me. They help me.

It is reassuring to me that relatives are helping her. Relatives visiting could be a reference to me, but in the context of the Other World of which she has spoken, it could refer to relatives who have passed over and be further evidence that she is nearing the end of her life.

Me: *Which relatives visit you?*
No reply.

If it had been me visiting she would have said so, so I imagine she is talking about her deceased relatives.

I have noticed that when I ask Mum for information about something she has just said, she sometimes doesn't answer me. This is always when the answer could have come from the *other side*. In future, I will presume, if she doesn't answer me, that this is the reason.

Me: *When you leave, will you continue to help me?*
Mum: *I will help you to help yourself.*

What a thoughtful and intelligent answer. This is not what I would have expected from someone suffering from advanced Alzheimer's disease.

Mum: *I will fill both cheeks.*

I interpret this to be a metaphor for giving me plenty of good and nourishing things to say. So there is more to come?

Mum: *I am unwell but I don't have a temperature. I should have a temperature.*

Her words indicate that her vitality is very low and clearly she is aware of this.

Mum: *I don't like not having my teeth.*

She has some dentures although she still has some of her own teeth.

Me: *Don't worry. You are lovely as you are. What I see is your soul.*
Mum: *Do I have a soul?*

My heart reaches out to her. How could such a beautiful soul not know itself?

Mum was the daughter of a Church of Scotland minister and she is asking me if she has a soul! What an indictment of the Church. Given what Mum has been talking about, one would assume that she has a deep knowledge of spirituality and the soul. But her question shows that everything that she is expressing is direct experience rather than being learned, labelled and remembered.

Me: *Everyone has a soul. You are your soul, and you are a most beautiful soul, Mum. Thank you for what you are giving me.*
Mum: *It's precious, Margaret, and should not be ignored.*

She is aware of the importance of the things she is telling me. I am, too, and take her words very much to heart. I am pleased I am recording them.

Although she does not know she has a soul as such, she knows that what we are discovering together is important.

Mum: *I don't want to be in hospital. I want to get up and get dressed and get on.*
Me: *Do you want to get up now?*
Mum: *No, not now.*

I reflect on all the things Mum has said today. Is her passing going to happen this week? I feel tearful every time I think about the possibility.

Back at home with Dad. When I tell him what Mum said, he immediately expresses his own needs, feelings of vulnerability and thoughts about his death. Although in his nineties, he hasn't talked about this before. My parents have never really been able to hear or be there for each other because of their own overwhelming needs.

Dad: *Give me a pill. I want to end it now!*

We talk about death and venture into discussing his death. He isn't interested in the process of dying – he just wants it to be over quickly and painlessly, as it would be if he died in his sleep. He expresses his relief that I am going to stay for a few more days, as well as his worry that I am going to have to deal with

Mum's death and his death on my own. I assure him that I can cope with whatever comes about. Surprisingly, I do believe this.

Monday 20 October 2003

Mum is looking contented and sitting in a chair in her room. I am sitting close to her, holding her wafer-thin hand.

Mum: *You have loving eyes, soft brown. Love is passing between us.*
You are being a great help to me.
All good things come at the end.

This is a very loving moment and I, too, feel love passing between us – the feeling is mutual. I have noticed that Mum has become very sensitive to what I am feeling, even when I am not saying anything, and this is enabling us to be closer. She is talking again about dying and every time she does I feel upset. I am stroking her.

Mum: *I will be around for a very long time. I will come to you, visit you. You have such wisdom. You help Margaret.*

She says that she expects to be around for a very long time, but clearly not in this world. What, then, is she seeing in the future? It sounds to me as if what she is experiencing is coming from the Other World.

Thursday 23 October 2003

Mum is in her room, sitting up in bed and looking reflective.

Mum: *These are very precious moments, Margaret.*

As she repeats this many times, I feel time is slowing down. Beautiful!

Mum: *I'm coming and going, can't remember.*
Thank you for keeping things moving along.

The decline in her memory is becoming more noticeable. By listening, respecting what she is saying and responding to it, I am helping her to stay connected to her worlds. I am glad she is appreciating this; it encourages me to continue on the same course.

Me: *Thank you for sharing your wisdom with me.*
Mum: *You can tell others.*
Me: *Thank you, I certainly will.*

This is clear confirmation of her wish that I share this information with you.

Mum: *I see tears.*

I don't have any now but later my tears come.

Mum: [Looks perplexed] *Don't cry.*
[Emphatically] *We are learning we're immortal, Margaret. I will be around. I'll flutter around you.*

Yes, this is what she is starting to show me on our Heart and Soul Journey: *we are immortal.* I need time and space to absorb this fully. What a wonderful message.

This is Mum's second reference to fluttering around me, and confirms my interpretation that she is thinking of herself as an energy form.

I have noticed recently that Mum has developed a repetitive habit of closing her eyes and moving her head from side to side, at the same time rubbing her nose and brow up and down. As she does this, little adjustments to the muscles in her face change her expression, but she does not say anything. I have come to realize that she does this when she is processing thoughts. Her memory is failing noticeably and I am trying to catch her thoughts before they disappear. So I wait until she stops moving, then immediately ask her what she is thinking, hoping it is still in her mind.

Mum: *You are mature. It is good of you to be with me just now. I'm remembering all my life: hobbled feet, little blobs, you and Fiona* [my deceased sister].
[Touching her heart] *William* [my dad] *and I will have coaching. How is William?*

'I'm remembering all my life': is this a *life review*, something that is commonly reported by people who've had a near death experience (NDE)? People who've had an NDE often say that they saw, during the time when they were clinically dead, their whole life passing before them. Does this mean Mum is going to die very soon?

'Hobbled feet' refers to the practice of tying together an animal's feet (usually a horse's), to restrict its movement. I interpret 'hobbled feet' as Mum's metaphor for her life that has been so restricted. What an accurate and sad statement – it makes me want to weep.

'Little blobs' sounds to me like my sister and me when we were embryos in her womb. How beautiful! How perfect!

It is true that Mum and Dad would benefit from coaching, but coaching is a fairly contemporary term, so I am surprised she has used it. Where did that come from?

Mum: *I'm trying to map out my brain.*
She repeats this a few times.
Where I'm going I will have your long hair. It's soft.

I am taken aback by this pronouncement. Again, I could dismiss it as her mind wandering, but 'I'm trying to map out my brain' is a conscious, complex mental activity. She knows she is going somewhere although she doesn't know where. She also has a vision of how her hair will be when she is there. When she was a young girl she had long hair. Is she talking about another

Other World that she has spoken about. Where am I? Where is Margaret? I am curious and keep these seeds in mind to see how they might develop.

Mum: *Which eye is dominant?*
Me: *Your left eye.*

My training in kinesiology and NLP enables me to notice eye dominance and interpret what it might mean for the person. When you observe someone, usually one eye appears more 'awake' than the other. The 'awake' eye is the dominant eye. Although eye dominance is more or less consistent, it can change temporarily as a result of certain kinds of activity. (There are also tests that can determine eye dominance.) I can see that Mum's left eye is dominant now.

Mum: *That is a good connection.*
Me: *Yes, I like it, too.*

Mum was right-handed and right-eye-dominant but this seems to have changed recently. I am left-handed and left-eye-dominant, hence the 'good connection' between us now. Incidentally, like many left-handed people, I am slightly dyslexic.

Mum: *Sometimes children die before their parents.*

This sounds like a remembrance of my sister Fiona.

After having been quite poorly, Mum is getting her will back. Every time I see her, as a matter of course, I offer her water and on this occasion she refuses to drink it. We joke about her being a rebel.

Mum's comment about children dying before their parents brings back poignant and very painful memories of 15 May 1999, when I gave permission for the doctors to turn off my sister's life support. My parents were anxiously waiting in a family room at the hospital and I remember telling them what was going to happen, then helping them as they staggered along the corridor, deeply distressed, toward the Intensive Care Unit to see their daughter for the last time. They were too upset to stay. A few minutes later the machines stopped. All was silent. Fiona had passed away and was at peace.

Saturday 25 October 2003

Mum is in her room, sitting up in bed and looking and sounding stronger.

Mum: *I can become unconscious, like having an operation with an anaesthetic, and get away from everything, then come back. I do it often.*

She is telling me that she has control over her state and can choose to be in a better place, maybe the Other World, and is doing this of her own volition. The medical view would be that this is a strategy someone suffering from depression might use to escape from the situation. But Mum has never described doing this before, so I think this strategy is new and clearly very effective.

Mum: *I love to flow ... the oceans, water. I do that often.*
Me: *That sounds wonderful, Mum.*

We live in an ocean of universal energy and when we are connected with it, we can sense that and 'go with the flow'. When Mum described how she could get away from everything and come back, I wondered if, in fact, her mind was leaving her physical body and going out into another dimension.

Mum: [Still in the flow of cosmic consciousness] *People matter. Everyone in the world matters!*

This is a wonderful universal thought and not the kind of statement Mum would have made earlier in her life, when she was operating at the level of individual consciousness. I wonder if this is a thought from the Other World.

Mum: *I try to remember my thoughts and can't.*
Me: *Don't worry Mum. We can just be.*
Mum: *You give me a feeling of calm, Margaret.*
Me: *I'm glad to hear that, Mum.*
Mum: *I'm breaking the flow but you have lovely teeth.*

She is aware of changing the direction of our conversation and seems intent on admiring my teeth. I have noticed that Mum pays me lots of compliments, particularly to do with my face, eyes and teeth. This is probably because she is focused, when we are talking, on this part of me and nothing else. So although it might seem that she is saying nice things to me to try to please me, I don't believe this is the case. She is saying exactly what she is seeing, without filtering her thoughts before she speaks like we do.

Mum: *I need to resolve some things with William.*
Me: *What things?*
Mum: *He doesn't feel deeply. I sometimes feel ...*

She tenses as she says this so I hold her and she immediately relaxes.

Dad, in common with most Scottish men of his generation, keeps his emotions well under control, while Mum is clearly looking for depth, meaning and connection on all levels. He visits her regularly but finds the care home a deeply depressing place, full of old people – not like him at ninety-two! As Mum's Alzheimer's progresses, he understands her even less than before and, being impatient by nature, his visits are always brief. As soon as he arrives he looks as if he is ready to leave.

I want to help her to relax.

Me: *All you do is take a big, big sigh and relax.*

She does it.

Mum: *Yes, it is so simple. Just like that.*
You look pensive tonight, Margaret.
The eyes. I can tell everything through the eyes, every expression, every feeling. This is good. These times together are helping us both.

This is true and confirms what my psychic friend conveyed to me.

When Mum looks at me with a long, unfaltering gaze, as she does frequently, I sense she can tell everything about me. We are all familiar with the expression, 'The eyes are the windows to the soul.'

Mum: [Playfully] *I'm a naughty girl. I dance.*
Me: *It's wonderful to dance, Mum.*

I am playing a CD of *Clair de Lune* and dancing around the room for her – and for me. I am glad that she is experiencing dancing through me. I just pray that no one will come in and see me! Staff members always knock first so I hope I will have time to regain my composure if this happens.

Later that evening, back at home with Dad, I think about the things Mum said to me about their relationship. I want to talk to him about it. I am aware that they have unresolved issues and I would like them to find reconciliation before the end of their lives. I struggle to find a way to open the conversation and make several abortive attempts, but he quickly moves the conversation on to something else. This clearly is a no-go area.

Sunday 26 October 2003

Mum is in her room in bed, very tired and sleepy. I am particularly conscious of how busy I have become, travelling up and down so much.

Mum: *I'm bored with life. My eyes are dull.*

This is true. How sad! This is why I am spending time with her. There is not much that she can do now.

Mum: *Your teeth, are they all right?*

How did she know I have been having problems with my teeth? She is psychic! This is a clear example of her ESP.

Mum: *You have a well-proportioned face. Lovely.* .

I am massaging her feet and stroking her gently.

Mum: *Very important, good. You have hot hands. Will you remember me?*
Me: *Of course I will remember you, Mum. How could I not? You are part of me. And I will remember what you are teaching me, especially about being loving.*
Mum: [Emphatically] *Love is what it is.*

Reflecting on love and Mum's profound statement, I think of her favourite hymn:

> O love that will not let me go,
> I rest my weary soul in thee:
> I give thee back the life I owe,
> That in thine ocean depths its flow
> May richer, fuller be.
>
> George Mattheson

Me: *Yes, you are right about love, Mum.*
Mum: *When I move where will I go, Margaret?*

This is the *big* question and of course I don't know. I have to think quickly on my feet. Her question confirms that she is talking from this world, yet other things she has said recently suggest she is also dipping into the Other World.

Me: *Where would you like to go?*
Mum: *Float, that would be lovely, to float.*
Me: *You could have a little floating experience now, if you like.*

The notion of floating comes naturally to Mum as a dancer, so it is understandable that she wants to enjoy this sensation, albeit through different means. Floating is also the kind of experience people have reported when leaving their body during NDEs or when astral travelling. I take her through a short guided visualization of floating.

After this we both close our eyes and are silent for a minute or two, then:

Mum: *I need to move my head so that I can breathe properly.*

Just before she said this, I was feeling a pain in the front of my neck that I knew wasn't mine – an example of my kinaesthetic sensitivity or clairsentience.

Mum: [Emphatically] *Wisdom, that's important.*

I am updating my list of the things that she is telling me are important.

Mum: *I want one hour of piano lessons. You must go to your family.*
       Kathleen, I haven't seen her for a long time.

Mum sounds a little confused, which could be due to a lack of oxygen as a result of her restricted breathing. Her thoughts could be coming from memories of her childhood. Kathleen is the name of her sister who died twenty-six years ago. She and Mum had piano lessons together as children. If this is a past memory that she is experiencing now, it demonstrates how she can slip almost seamlessly into a different time.

Monday 3 November 2003

Mum is in her room sitting up in bed, looking reflective.

Me: *Hello Mum. It's lovely to see you. How are you? How are*
      you feeling?
Mum: *Average, Margaret.*
      I feel I have no past, present or future.
Me: *What is that like?*
No reply.

This is a description of nothingness and sounds to me like a state
of total dissociation. Maybe she is articulating what people with
Alzheimer's experience at times. Or maybe she is in an Other
World, in which time as we know it does not exist.

Mum: *I can't remember – two prongs, the wrong word. I still*
      have two tickets. I want to be able to remember still.

'Two tickets' suggests two more opportunities. Numbering
like this is a code commonly used by people at the end of life
to indicate the options they have left. Thankfully, despite her
repeated announcements about dying, it seems she is not going
just yet.

Tuesday 4 November 2003

Mum is relaxed in bed. She seems to be having thoughts but
can't remember what they are.

Mum: *Meridian, is that the right word? Channels of thought.*

In acupuncture meridians are invisible channels through which
chi energy flows. So this is an interesting application of the
term 'meridian' and an example of how people with Alzheimer's,
when they can't find the word they want to use, often substitute
another word that has the same or similar meaning. Both

'meridian' and 'channels of thought' have energy associations. I wonder if this is what she means.

Me: *Go with the flow.*

Mum likes this and I tell her I will send her the 'Go with the Flow' greetings card I have designed.

Mum's voice is so soft and gentle it makes me aware that my own voice could be warmer, softer and more expressive. Also, she is giving me very direct, positive feedback, such as, 'You have beautiful eyes.' I could respond more in the same way and be more direct with her. I commit to doing so.

Saturday 15 November 2003

I have been busy catching up with my life in London: meeting with friends, seeing clients, teaching, walking on the Heath, swimming, going to the ballet, attending talks and doing all the other things I enjoy doing when I am in the city. I even found time to go to the dentist and he confirmed the tooth problem Mum had mentioned in one of her psychic moments.

When I return I find Mum in her room sitting in a chair and looking bright. I notice that she is wearing an unfamiliar striped blouse that has found its way into her wardrobe, as happens in care homes. I haven't seen her for a little while and am very happy to be with her again.

Me: *Hello Mum. It's lovely to see you again. How are you?*
        How are you feeling?
Mum: *Fine, thank you, Margaret.*
        I've never seen such love coming from anyone's eyes.
Me: *That is so lovely, Mum. You are responsible for that.*

I feel full of love. This is at the heart of our journey together. It shows how we are both responding to each other's loving feelings.

Sunday 16 November 2003

Mum is in bed.

Mum: *I need a friend.*
Me: *What kind of friend?*

In the context of everything she has been talking about, I interpret this as a spiritual request.

Mum: *I don't know. I need to move on and can't.*

My heart goes out to her – I understand what she is talking about.

Mum: *Emily and me, she is not ready, she needs more. But don't worry about that now.*

Emily has never talked about her granny dying and I don't think she wants to contemplate this. She has had to come to terms with her mum dying. My dear mum needs to move on but Emily is not ready to deal with her granny's death. I think Mum might be holding on until she is.

Mum: *I want to be fit.*
Me: *You will be, Mum. You will be fit. You will be able to move freely and dance to your heart's content. You will get whatever you want. You will get whatever you think, whatever you imagine.*
Mum: *I'll remember that. I know what you are talking about, what you mean.*

Amazing, utterly amazing! I know about how we create our reality because I have learned about this and often experienced it in my own life. Mum has not had such exposure but nevertheless she knows intuitively. This is a function of the soul. It is this kind of symbiosis of the heart and soul that is enabling our journey and 'keeping things moving along'.

Mum: *I need to position myself for you so that I can be useful.*

She has made another reference to 'position' (she also spoke about this on 23 October). She is thinking of me again. How nice to know that she wants to be useful to me. I know in my heart that she will be, and am deeply touched. I am reminded again that my psychic friend told me that Mum and I are going to help each other. Clearly, we are.

Mum: *The treatment has ended. There will be no more.*
      My head is not attached to my body.

Help! She looks the same to me, but her perception of herself is suddenly very different. What she is describing about her head not being attached to her body sounds to me like an out-of-body experience. It suggests a state of total dissociation and could be a sensation people with Alzheimer's disease experience when parts of their brain aren't functioning. But it is surprising that she can articulate it. She has described being in a dissociated state before, and has been telling me in this world about her experiences in the Other World. This suggests she is indeed working between two worlds.

Mum: *I need to say goodbye to Emily before I leave.*

Tears fill my eyes again at the thought of her leaving and I know my niece will be deeply upset, too.

She said, 'The treatment has ended.' Is this the end, I wonder? I reflect on the last three months, on our intimate sharing and on the beautiful symbiosis that has developed between us. Mum has told me the most wonderful things about life and death with an authority that is without question. I desperately want to tell everyone about these revelations but what Mum has said needs to be understood as a whole, otherwise it could sound insubstantial. Who can I tell? Who will believe me?

Clearly, I can't tell Dad. He goes to church on Sunday and if the minister were to repeat the things Mum has said he might believe him, but neither Mum nor I have that authority in his eyes. I could try to tell my son, Paul, but I can't tell him everything as it would take too long and I suspect his rational mind will view a brief version of events with scepticism. He knows how difficult Mum has been in the past, so it would be hard for him to comprehend such a complete turnaround without witnessing it himself. My niece Emily is a pragmatist, so there is no opportunity there. I have friends in London who would understand such things but they are far removed from the situation. I really want people who know Mum to know what wisdom she possesses and to celebrate this. So here I am, on my own and no one with whom I can share my soul's excitement.

Monday 17 November 2003

Mum is sitting in her chair, leaning forward and looking slightly anxious, not relaxed. I hug her gently and she relaxes. She starts talking about Emily.

Mum: *There is wisdom in the cracks.*

This is another beautiful metaphor. What a poetic way of putting it. I am aware of this, too.

Mum: [Talking about me, emphatically] *You must do what you want. Do you understand that?*

This is very pertinent. I neglect my creativity at considerable cost to myself.

There is a lesson here for all of us. Doing what we love helps us to become more who we really are, and in turn this helps others.

Mum: *I must give you a date. I will do that. I don't know yet. When should I sleep?*

I am so relieved that she is going to give me notice. I want to be with her at the end.

Mum: *I have access to a, like a first-aid box. I can go to it at any time and get whatever I need. It is wonderful ... an injection in my brain.*
Me: *That's absolutely amazing, Mum! How do you do that?*
No reply.

She makes it sound so simple. Maybe it is and you just do it. It sounds like something she is initiating and is able to access from the Other World.

However, 'an injection in my brain' – I fear we are approaching the end of any meaningful conversation and that this could mark the conclusion of our journey together as we have known it. I feel upset and very sad at this prospect.

Friday 5 December 2003

It is a couple of weeks since I have seen Mum and I am feeling a little apprehensive. Are we still going to be able to communicate in the way we have in the past, given the bizarre things she was saying at the end of my last visit?

It is morning and Mum is in her room, sitting in a chair. She is bright but has a rattling cough.

Me: *Hello Mum. It's lovely to see you. How are you? That is quite a cough you have.*

64

Mum: *Average.*
  I've got to finish for Margaret.

I know what she means but don't want to talk about it.

Mum: *I had the two tests. I didn't do anything underhand.*
Me: *What were the two tests?*
No reply.
Me: *What were the results?*
Mum: *Good.*
Me: *That's good. You're doing well, Mum.*

As this information seems to be coming from her Other World, are these tests that her soul has chosen to undertake in order to be purified so that she can evolve spiritually? People like Diana Cooper who channel information from the Other World say there are seven initiations on the spiritual path, each of which involves learning and tests. The seven initiations relate to the seven levels of energy that surround the body. The first initiation involves the first level of the energy field, the one closest to the physical body, and can result in a spiritual awakening. The second relates to the emotional body and involves learning to taking charge of the emotions. My observations are that Mum has indeed passed both these tests.

Mum: [Emphatically] *These are wonderful moments. Remember them and feel them.*

Thank goodness, she is still connecting with me and in a beautiful way. How wise she is. It is feeling rather than thinking that matters. I stop now and feel this.

Good feelings produce endorphins in the brain that in turn create more good feelings. It is a very positive cycle.

Mum: *I don't want it* [death] *but it has got to be. I need to get my energies in the right position. I am getting everything ready in a position for starting.*

Well, there is no denial of death here. She is taking a positive course of action. A few weeks ago she said the treatment had ended, and now she is talking about getting ready for starting. This sounds like the end of one stage and the beginning of a new one, possibly the next initiation, indicating that there is indeed a process. Again, she is talking about being in the right position, showing me that she is fully aware, at some level, of what she is doing. I am both curious and amazed.

Mum: *Special people, special places, special things to say – but I don't know what they are.*

This sounds like an awareness she has gained while visiting the Other World that she is unable to articulate here in the physical world.

Me: *Don't worry.*

I want to reassure her that she shouldn't regret not being able to tell me.

Mum: *A preview, peace and quiet.*

As she says this I, too, sense peace and quiet and this gives me comfort.

All the things she is saying are glimpses of the Other World and related to passing on. This preview of the Other World is very positive, as is the look of peace in her face.

Mum: *I'm happy. Things are working out as they are meant to. There is extra time.*

I am so happy, too. She knows how things are meant to be. This kind of knowing is coming from somewhere else. After all the rehearsals and near misses it does seem as though we have been given the gift of extra time together. I am immensely grateful for it and cannot help but wonder if she has requested the 'extra time', or somehow or other realizes it has been granted. Either way, it gives us each a chance to experience more of the good feelings, and allow any lingering bad memories from the past to melt away.

Mum: *What if it doesn't work out? I am an anxious person. I will put it in your calendar. I haven't done it yet.*

Suddenly she has snapped back into this world again, still haunted by the old underlying anxiety that has plagued her throughout her life. Despite her obvious unease about timing, I'm relieved that she is intending to let me know about her death in advance. As we become closer, so does our need to let go of one another as gently as possible. I never dreamed I would feel this way about Mum.

Saturday 6 December 2003

Mum is sitting up in her bed, looking eager to talk.

Mum: *The inspectors came to see me. I usually know when they're coming. Kathleen* [her deceased sister] *is very polite to them. They come for Emily. They ask me questions – straightforward questions. I can answer. They're very reassuring.*

'I usually know when they're coming', suggests that the inspectors have been before, possibly when she reported having had the two tests.

'They come for Emily' indicates that the inspectors are helping Emily, possibly through Mum.

Her reference to her late sister Kathleen implies an after-death contact. She has made references to Kathleen and deceased relatives in the spirit world before.

This latest report from Mum confirms my recent thoughts that she is, unknowingly yet very naturally, acting as a medium, channelling information from the Other World to this world and perhaps back again.

Mum: *I'm at peace in myself.*
Me: *That is so good to know, Mum. I feel the same way when
     we are together like this.*
Mum: *You will live a long life, if you want a long life.*

Well, this is good to know. I have a choice. That is very reassuring
and I will remember it when I am fretting unnecessarily about
some minor complaint, as I sometimes do.

Sunday 7 December 2003

Mum is in her room, sitting in a chair and looking bright.

Me: *Hello Mum. How are you? How are you feeling? You're
     looking bright.*
Mum: *I'm fine, thank you, Margaret.*

This is a positive response. She is clearly having a good day.
    I read Mum a very thoughtful letter that she wrote to me
many years ago. Afterwards, I discover that my audio recorder
has mysteriously failed to record, despite indicating that it
was functioning normally. Thankfully, I am also making
written notes.

Mum: *These are precious moments. You have lovely teeth. You
     are a lovely girl. You have helped me to feel happy and
     contented. All I need is your name and date on a piece
     of paper.*
     *I want Margaret to have understanding. She needs
     understanding.*

I am so glad I am helping her.
    We all need understanding – Margaret and me included.
Growing up too quickly has made it hard for me to show my
needs at times. But despite our battles in the past Mum can now
see the vulnerability that lies behind my strong exterior. I cannot
keep the tears at bay.

Mum: *I am helping Emily. She is funny. I don't talk to her about exams. Her thoughts are simple ... in the pages. We* [Mum and I] *bridge the age gap. Don't be worried, there is nothing wrong.*

She hasn't seen Emily recently so it appears I guessed correctly about my niece receiving help from the Other World through Mum. 'In the pages' sounds like a book of some kind. It would seem I am some kind of bridge, too, and I am very happy to take on this role.

Tuesday 23 December 2003

I am back in Scotland for Christmas and delighted to be here with the family, but I am soon shocked to find Mum in her room looking utterly abandoned. Her hair is not washed and she seems to be sorely neglected. This has never happened before and I can only surmise that there is a staff shortage and that the care assistants are busy with all the extra arrangements for Christmas. Paul, my son, is with me. He, too, notices Mum's dishevelled appearance.

Paul is my only son, Mum's only grandson, and Emily's cousin. He is twenty-five years old and lives in London, where he is studying. As a child he spent many happy summer holidays at my parents' house. Far from the confines of the big city, he and Emily loved playing on the beach in the bracing sea air. He is close to both my parents and enjoys being with them and his cousin.

Me: *Hello Mum. It's lovely to see you. How are you? How are you feeling?*
Mum: *Fair.*
It's sad but it has to be. I want it to be right. It was clear and now it is not.

So something is not sitting right with her. What might that be?

Paul: *What do you want to be right, Granny?*
No reply.

As I have already noted, when Mum doesn't reply it seems to indicate that information is coming to her from the Other World. So her words do not just reflect distress in the physical world.

Mum: *Emily. I've taken off her straitjacket and now she is free. Emily is a nice girl. She is straightforward.*

Mum's comments about Emily are very perceptive and positive. They show that she is helping Emily, albeit from the Other World.

Mum: *William. I want him to know where he is going. He has lessons to learn.*

I am touched by Mum's concern for Dad. I love him dearly too and I want him to find the same kind of resolution that she is finding. He doesn't have her insight. It is becoming more obvious to me that she is consciously working between two worlds, helping Emily, Dad and me.

I am noticing that Mum is giving me an increasing amount of information from the Other World. I am so glad that I chose to travel with her on this path and that I have been keeping an open mind about what she says, no matter how strange it might sound at the time. Had I not done this, I believe none of this privileged information would have been forthcoming.

I am also convinced of the importance of being Mum's scribe, and I have settled into this role over the last four months. Keeping a record of our conversations and my thoughts is helping me to stay connected to her in a meaningful way, and taking time to reflect is deepening my understanding of the mystical process that is unfolding.

I return to her concern for Dad.

Me: *Can I help you and Dad?*
Mum: *No.*
       My thinking is confused. The fall I had in the summer affected me.

I wasn't informed that she had had a fall in the summer, but that doesn't mean she didn't have one. These things are supposed to be recorded in the care-home log and conveyed to a relative. Perhaps it was a fall on another plane.

Mum: *Our connection will continue.*

I wonder what timeframe she has in mind. Is she referring to our connection in this world or in the Other World, after she has passed on?

Mum: *Do you want to continue to ask me questions? How the four parts of my brain are connected?*
Me: *Yes please!*

Wow! How fascinating! I am impressed that she initiated this conversation. But just as I am going to ask her about her brain, she moves on swiftly to something else. Damn it, I really want to find out about this.

She is right about the four parts of the brain. But how does she know how the parts of her brain are connected?

At times, it might seem that I missed an opportunity to ask Mum a pertinent question, but I had learned not to interrupt her when she was in a stream of consciousness as to do so could bring the process to an abrupt halt, because she was often unable to remember what she had just said. I make a mental note that I need to change my strategy and be quicker off the mark in future, so that I can catch these fleeting thoughts before they disappear.

Mum: [Moving on without hesitation] *Paul is nice.*

I notice that she is talking about Paul in the third person, too, despite his presence. Is she seeing Paul in an energetic form? I am wondering if she is in a dissociated state, if everything and everyone seem a step removed to her?

She has made meaningful comments about Emily, Dad, Paul and me. It is Christmas and we are around; it is as if she is conducting a review of all the family members.

Mum: *I am well. It's my nerves.*

So this state she is in seems to be a reminder of her lifelong struggle with her nerves. Poor Mum.

Christmas Day 2003

What a transformation from a couple of days ago. Mum now looks fine and composed. Her hair is lovely and she is wearing a beautiful printed blouse and pleated skirt that I bought for her. She spends part of the day in the care home joining in the festivities there, and after that we bring her round in a wheelchair to our house to enjoy the family celebrations with us. It is good that we can do this so seamlessly – a real gift.

Mum seems reflective but is present in her own quiet and gracious way. Being at home together as a family feels very loving and warm.

When it is time to return to the care home, and I roll the wheelchair along in the cold and the dark, I find it really painful and sad to have to take her away from the heart of the family and her home, but no words are spoken about this. We both know it must be. During this busy festive time there is no quiet time for Mum and me to connect in our special way in our sacred space. We must be content with the more public holiday affections.

Friday 26 December 2003

Mum is in her room, looking tired.

Mum: *I'm thinking about the move. I have to do this one on my own.*

I interpret this to be a move to the next phase, either in this life or passing from this world to the Other World. And yes, if the latter is the case, she has to do this one on her own.

Me: *You'll do it.*
Mum: *I'm doing all right. The keys to the house, anyone can come in.*

How fascinating. In dreams the house is often a symbol of the self. She is indeed open to all!

Mum: *Margaret is disconnected.*
Emily isn't home yet. She will be fine.
It's important to have a happy home.

Oops! Is Margaret disconnected? I must be if Mum says so. This may be due to all the Christmas activities. She is right: when other people are around I am unable to connect with her in the very intuitive and intimate way I do when we are on our own. I feel inhibited and imagine that even close family members will not understand what we are talking about.

I think the meaning of 'home' in Emily's case may have to do with being at home in herself.

As you are already aware, we as a family did not have a happy home, so Mum's statement 'It's important to have a happy home' may indicate a newly found realization following the healing times we have had over the last few months.

Saturday 27 December 2003

Mum is in her room and a care assistant brings a tray of tea and biscuits for us.

Mum: *It feels very homely.*

You're a lovely girl, Margaret. So nice, there is something so nice about you.

We are chatting and Mum keeps looking to her right and staring into the distance. She says she sees a space but I can't see what she's talking about. From time to time she reports seeing a space like this. I imagine she is seeing some kind of energy that is simply not visible to me.

Mum: *Two keys so that I can come and go when I want to.*

Maybe she was seeing a space in another dimension. Her comment about the keys and coming and going suggests control and the choice to move back and forth between the two worlds.

Mum: *Emily and Margaret. Margaret has her freedom.*
Me: *Yes I have, Mum, and I thank you for helping me to find it.*

I imagine, when she talks about Margaret in my presence, that she is seeing me in her mind's eye.

Mum: *He doesn't mean it but William forgets I have a conscience. I'm keeping in touch.*
Me: *I don't think he resents anything now.*
Mum: *I think he realizes it's too much together.*

I am guessing she means they have weathered too much together to turn away now.

Me: *He is really trying hard to connect with you.*
Mum: *All that richness is available.*

So true and so beautifully put. As she already told me, she is open to everyone.

Me: *Thank you.*
Mum: *Don't say it so reluctantly.*

74

Oops! She can be very direct. I think that my defence of Dad may have reminded her of the past when I frequently supported him at her expense. Clearly, in just two words, I slipped back into that old frame of relating to her. Mum has become extremely sensitive to nuances of expression and responds immediately to what she is picking up.

Me: *Thank you.* [Emphatically] *Thank you very much, Mum.*
Mum: [After a long pause] *The stillness of deep love, I can't find*
          words to describe it.
          Precious moments. I want you to remember the
          good times.

How utterly wonderful! These are words from the heart and soul of someone who has transcended life as you and I know it, and found the true meaning of love. I feel overwhelmed and silent tears are welling up in me.

Mum: *I need to be in the right position.*

Again, Mum is talking about the right position. This must be really important.

Mum: *Who will look after the music?*
Me: *Emily will.*

There is a history of music in Mum's family. Her mother, sister and she all played the piano and sang in choirs. My niece Emily is the one who has carried on this tradition. She has a lovely voice and is also a member of a choir. For years this has been an important part of her life.

Mum: *I've got my brain organized.*
Me: *How do you do that?*
Mum: *I think of something, anything, and take it from*
          there. Television.

Mum doesn't normally watch TV, so I am wondering if she is talking about an inner television – or tele-vision. Could this be a portal through which the information from the Other World is coming to her? This sounds like the way some psychics describe their experience of channelling. They say they see with their mind's eye, their third eye, something like a TV screen, through which they can view and listen to the information that streams in. Mum is also telling me that she is choosing what she wants from her tele-vision.

Sunday 28 December 2003

Mum is in her room. She has a slight cold and her eyes look distant. I notice that she is working hard, turning her head from side to side as she does when she is thinking and processing information. Then she stops and stares intently at a particular spot in the room.

Me: *You're looking over there. What do you see, Mum?*
Mum: *A little gap. Do you not notice it?*
Me: *No.*
Mum: *I don't know what is over there.*

This could be a visual disturbance, commonly reported in people with Alzheimer's. However, I am keeping an open mind. She may be perceiving something like an energy that I can't see. I wish I were more sensitive to these energies.

Mum: *How to get the programme for Emily. Margaret will record it. She does everything like that.*

Was she seeing something about Emily's programme in the 'little gap'? I promise to follow up and record the programme for Emily. This may involve taking note of the programme and communicating it in some form to Emily.

Mum: *I am getting the markers in place for the move. The timer is to stop at 3pm. Make sure the radiators are on. When my friend goes I will give you the address. Time, there is not much time. Time is difficult. Time doesn't matter. We will work it out. It will be fine.*

Mum sounds quite confused but, reading between the lines, there are some messages with a common theme here. Move, keys, new address, time – all are indicators of moving on. Thankfully, she is reassuring me it will be fine. I note that she is telling me that time doesn't matter, something many sages and transcendental philosophers tell us.

Mum: *These are precious moments. You're a lovely girl, Margaret.*
You have a good character. Your teeth are lovely. Just one pocket of resistance, it's medical.
Me: [Quickly and worriedly] *What is it?*
Mum: *I can't remember. I'm trying to work it out. I can't get the words. I can … it isn't serious. I think there's one little pocket of resistance. It's a medical thing.*

Monday 29 December 2003

Mum is in her room, looking bright and very cosy. She is in a thoughtful mood.

Mum: *Avisandum.*
Me: *I've never heard of that word. What does it mean, Mum?*
Mum: *It means a curtailment to the next day. Take it to avisandum.*

I looked it up and, sure enough, it is a Scottish legal term meaning 'further consideration'. Where did that come from? It sounds to me that this information is coming to her from somewhere else.

Mum: *There is no place for the wrinkles.*

I think this could be a metaphor for the need for everything to be fresh, visible and out in the open. She certainly is taking this approach.

Mum: *Your eyes spell peace.*
Me: *Thank you, Mum. I feel peaceful when I am with you.*

Mum looks as if she is beating time and I ask her what she is doing.

Mum: *Trying to think of a tune. Time three-four rhythm. I'm stupid.*
Me: *Oh no, you are certainly not stupid, Mum. You are extremely intelligent.*
Mum: *Intelligent. That gives me lots of help to get over the transition period that is not easy.*

I can tell my acknowledgement and validation of her has boosted her confidence. She recognizes that she is in a process, a transition from one stage to another and possibly from one world to another, and I'm glad my reassurance is helping to support her in this.

Me: *You are doing everything exactly as it should be done and with such intelligence. You have opened yourself up completely.*

The look on Mum's face confirms how pleased she is to be given this affirmation. It is boosting her confidence.

Mum: *I've got to wait until some messages come through. I'm trying to get everything organized so that I can relax.*

The reference to messages coming through might be considered by the medical profession to be a symptom of schizophrenia.

Given Mum's declaration a few weeks ago that she was receiving information from the inspectors, I believe she is, albeit unknowingly, acting as a medium or channel. She is being given instructions from the other side, from the Other World.

Mum: *It will come right in the end. When you came up there was a certain amount of disconnection. I want to make it right.*

Although she is very forgetful now, she remembers that I had difficulties in joining her in her world with all the people around over Christmas, and she is determined to get our connection back. But I wonder how she remembered this when she has difficulty in recalling what she has just said? I imagine the feeling she had then is coming back to her.

I am massaging her feet very gently, as I often do.

Mum: *I like when you do both feet. It makes a complete circuit of what I want.*

She is right about the complete circuit in terms of the nerve endings, meridians and flow of energy. I am so glad she is benefiting from it.

We are talking about our time together and appreciating all the incredible things that are happening.

Mum: *It will never leave you. It's part of you.*

Oh, how lovely! I know this is true but it is nevertheless reassuring to have Mum tell me.

Mum: *It will come soon. I'll work it out.*
Three-four rhythm.
We're piloting ideas. We're pioneers.

Me: *Yes we are and it's exciting. You're teaching me the things I've always wanted to know and more. This is a truly wonderful gift, Mum. Thank you.*

Mum: *It won't leave you. Tears will come soon.*

And tears did come. And they still come. When I feel something very precious, deep inside, I have a feeling of filling up and tears are my way of expressing this. They are not tears of sadness. This is a feeling and not a thought, so it does not need to be translated into words. It is beyond words.

Wednesday 31 December 2003

I am in London and on the phone to Mum, something I try to do every day when I am away. This helps to keep the connection between us.

Mum: *When I am in this system it is difficult to ...*
Me: *What system?*
Mum: *This x-ray system.*

Mum is describing an invisible system but exactly which one is not clear to me. Is this a metaphor for the telephone or is this 'x-ray system' a description of how she views the Other World?

Although speaking on the phone is no substitute for being with her, I can't be in Scotland 24/7 and remain totally present for her. I need to recharge my batteries. So although out of sight temporarily, the phone ensures I am not out of mind, and I love hearing her voice, too. I always end my calls by saying, 'I'm sending you a *big* hug and a *big* kiss.'

PORTAL TO THE OTHER WORLD

'I can go there and everything is just how I want it.'
Pat

2004

While in London I get together again with my psychic friend. A spontaneous reading ensues. He is told: 'Maggie is angelic and has come down to help.' Well, I am no angel, so I understand this to be more a term of endearment. My friend says that my work will change as a result of my journey with Mum, and I can already sense a shift occurring. Regarding Mum he reports, 'It is possible a "new package" will come for her'; I don't know what that means.

Sunday 18 January 2004

I have been away for a few weeks and am back. Mum is in her room, sitting in her chair.

Me: *Hello Mum. It's lovely to see you. How are you? You look lovely and cosy.*
Mum: *Average.*
        Emily has her tele-vision and can listen.

My interpretation is that Emily, as a result of Mum's intervention and 'the inspectors', can now access her inner senses, the part of her that has wisdom and knows. How wonderful! I wonder how she might be experiencing this? Might she be hearing her inner voice? Emily might not even be aware of it, but having spent time with her recently I can confirm that something very positive is starting to happen to her.

Mum: *Little things to remember, little things to forget. Patience. How am I going to finish this? I should just let it happen.*
Me: *Everything is just as it's meant to be.*

I really believe this.

Later:

Mum: *I need to have a tooth out.*

Her comment prompts me to tell the nursing staff to make an appointment with the dentist. Things like dental check-ups tend to be forgotten unless a specific need arises, as is the case now.

Mum: *Where am I?*
Me: *You are in the care home Mum, right next door to your home. I am with you and everything is just as it should be.*

This is the first time she has been confused like this. I wonder if she has an infection in her tooth and if that is affecting her brain. Who knows how long it's been like this.

A photo showing her house and the care home right next door is pinned up on the wall of her room. I bring it over to her and we talk about this close connection.

Monday 19 January 2004

I am talking with Mum in her room.

Mum: *I hear the tune, work it out in bars and put it into words.*

Although we are not aware of it, different parts of the brain are involved in processing incoming information and this does happen in a sequence. It is possible that she is more aware of this now that Alzheimer's has slowed down her thought process. Another possibility is that she now has to process information in a different, more complex way. Does she have to go through the complicated process she describes in order to speak?

Alternatively, is she hearing frequencies from the Other World and decoding them? It seems to me, from all the different kinds of experiences she is having, that Mum is indeed progressing from the physical to the non-physical, from this world to the Other World.

Mum: *I didn't want to be anaesthetized.*

She is saying this in the past tense, though she has not yet been to the dentist. In the past, whenever she visited the dentist, she would request not to have injections or be anaesthetized. She didn't like to be out of control. I wonder if something happened in her brain yesterday to lead her to ask, 'Where am I?'

Thursday 5 February 2004

I haven't seen Mum for a couple of weeks. She is in her room and I sit down right next to her and hold her hand.

Me: *Hello Mum. It's lovely to see you. How are you? How are you feeling?*
Mum: *Average.*
You have lovely teeth, a lovely face – a healthy looking face.
Me: *Thank you, Mum. I have you and Dad to thank for my healthy genes.*

The Gift of Alzheimer's

You will have noticed that Mum pays me lots of compliments. These are not confined to me. The care assistants and nursing staff also get showered in compliments like this, but working with people who have Alzheimer's they are accustomed to it.

I tell her about a dream I had about birth.

Mum: *We are all living in an Other World.*

This is another announcement about the Other World, which apparently includes the dream world.

Mum: *I don't want to make too many changes for Margaret.*
Margaret is a woman.

I wonder what changes she is talking about. Might they be changes to her or changes to me?

Mum: *It's nice we have parallel thoughts.*
Me: *Yes, it's good for both of us.*
Mum: *I can go there and everything is just how I want it.*

It's true – I have noticed how aligned our thoughts have become and how this is giving us a feeling of closeness.

I am assuming that 'there' is some level in the Other World. It could be what she accesses through what she calls 'television', as she recently reported being able to get what she wanted from it. As Mum is growing closer to the end of her life and her physical senses are atrophying, it seems that her inner senses are awakening.

Me: *Yes, Mum, you can have whatever you want. What you think is what you get.*
Mum: *These are good words.*

I have just made a really profound statement and she understands it completely.

existence in the Other World? I can see from her repetitive head movements that she is processing a lot of information.

She goes on to use the word 'temporal' and I ask her to explain what she means; in dementia people often have difficulty in finding the word to express a thought, although they can understand others. This does not seem to be what is happening in Mum's case.

Mum: *Temporal, meaning of this life.*
        [Slowly raising and observing her hand in front of her]
        My little wrist, silly.

My heart fills. She is looking intently at her old, very thin wrist and her bony hand with its slightly contracted fingers, and contemplating what she is seeing.

Me: *No Mum, not silly, definitely not silly.*
Mum: *My fingers, they are so thin. They won't be thin for long.*
        [Emphatically] *Death is nothing to be afraid of. I'm in no pain. I'm content.*
Me: *That is wonderful, absolutely wonderful, Mum.*

Again, I am stunned by her perception of death and the afterlife. She is describing a vision of herself in what I imagine to be the Other World and has a very positive perception of how she will be after she has left this world. Clearly, she is not afraid of dying.

I feel very reassured, not just for her, but also for myself and for all those who seek similar comfort.

Mum's precognition of death suggests that she has already visited the Other World or had a preview of her life there.

Having just heard Mum's words about eternal life, yet stuck in temporal time myself, I am thinking about my plans and the timing of my travel back to London. I reluctantly broach the subject with her.

Me: *I have a decision to make: to go tomorrow or to stay.*

Mum: *Stay. I'm not ready to go just yet. What do you think is happening to us, Margaret?*

We are both aware something very special is happening so I decide to rearrange my plans and stay for a few more days.

Me: *Our souls are helping each other, Mum.*

A psychic friend has told me that Mum and I are on this journey to help each other, and that Mum is going to raise me to a higher vibrational level. His reading was that Mum is slipping over to the other side and holding up a mirror for me to see. He said it was payback time for me, after having had such a difficult childhood. His words really resonated with me.

Mum: *My brain has cleared. The flu has lifted. I want to be in the right position. There is nothing else I can tell you. I've had three or four operations.*

Well, I didn't know anything about these operations, but she certainly seems in good form. It all sounds to me like a process. First, a number of operations on her mind to clear her brain. Then, getting into the right position – but the right position for what? Moving on to where?

If this is the end and she has nothing else to say to me then I have to accept it, but I will miss her uplifting messages. She has become the focus of my life. I would never have believed I would hear myself saying this about Mum, with whom I have had so many difficulties in the past.

I am thinking about all the things Mum has talked about today and I am feeling deeply moved.

Friday 24 October 2003

Mum is in her room, sitting up in bed. She is trembling and shaking. This is the first time I have seen her like this and it is very distressing.

Mum: *Held together.*

I am holding her firmly and stroking her lovingly. Soon she starts to calm down.

Mum: *Your hands are so hot.*

I wasn't trying to do anything and was unaware I had hot hands just then, though I first discovered this phenomenon when I started working with energy and healing in the early eighties. Healers often get hot hands when energy is flowing from the Source. It is important to emphasize that healers don't actually do anything other than focus their attention on the person, feel the connection, and let energy radiate and flow.

Mum: *Your teeth are so white. They are still good despite all the moves. You get a grip with your teeth. You have a lovely face. You have a well-proportioned face.*
Me: *Thank you, Mum.*

'Get a grip with your teeth' is, I think, another way of saying, 'get your teeth into something'. It's true. I do focus and get on with things.

Mum: *Where is Emily* [her granddaughter]*? What is she doing? Does she know I've had another operation?*
Me: *Emily is in Glasgow. She is working. She doesn't know about your special operations.*

Emily is Mum's only granddaughter, my sister Fiona's only child and my niece. In her early twenties, having found her own feet as an adult, she moved from my parents' house to Glasgow. For many years her passion in life has been to work in the media, particularly in television, and she continues to seek opportunities in this highly competitive field. She is twenty-nine now and often comes down to visit her grandparents at weekends.

Mum: *The people that matter: Margaret and Fiona. Have you seen Fiona?*
Me: *Mum, I know that you have just forgotten for the moment that Fiona passed on some years ago.*
Mum: *Oh yes, I forgot about that. It doesn't matter.*

Her remembrance of my sister is particularly touching. Since Fiona died four years ago, no one has spoken about her – it is as if she were better forgotten. But Mum has not forgotten her and neither have I.

After some conversation:

Me: *What is really important, Mum?*
Mum: *People.*

Mum was quite self-obsessed in the past, so this is a significant shift in her outlook.

I have my hands on her and am feeling the connection and our energies radiating and flowing.

Mum: *A rush of illuminations, lots of light.*

We pause and appreciate this experience together.

Mum: *Margaret left with something in her ear last night.*
Me: *What was that, Mum?*
Mum: *The things I told her.*

This is a great example of metaphor.

I have noticed that Mum has started referring to me in both the second and third person, as if I am two people. At times I am addressed directly as 'you' or as 'Margaret', and at others it is as though in her mind I exist alongside someone else called Margaret, like a double. At the beginning she said, *'It is difficult being ... working between two worlds.'* One world, presumably, is the physical world that she and I inhabit. And then there is the

Mum: *I'm happy living and just going on. We have help. I can't see it, but I know it is there.*

These are all very reassuring words to me. She is tuned into the Other World and I sense it too, but not as clearly as she does. So it seems that she is remaining here on the Earth plane, for the time being.

Friday 6 February 2004

Mum is in her room, sitting in a chair, leaning forward and watching a programme on TV – something she rarely does. Her hands and feet are very cold and I am warming them. It's a nature programme. It finishes and we start talking.

Mum: *I have courage.*
Me: *Yes Mum, you certainly do.*
Mum: *My dream: it's the climax. This is the end. It's peaceful. It's amazing, the thought process. I feel well. I haven't felt like this for a long time.*

I am amazed, too. What a positive message! It seems that Mum has faced her own death. What courage! I am filled with admiration.

I note the sequence: dream, end, peace, thought and, finally, feeling well. Two months ago Mum said, 'A preview, peace and quiet.' Now it seems her dream has taken her beyond that stage to the next one. I believe she may have gone to a higher level of consciousness in the spiritual plane, where thought is said to be all-important.

Mum: *I want to be in a position to help and care for you.*
Margaret put something in my gargle. My feet are dancing. I will dance.
Special moments. Loving being loved by you.

As Mum said earlier, 'Love is what it is.' How utterly lovely! I feel very present and full of gratitude when she says she wants to help and care for me. Because of her overwhelming needs, my needs didn't always come first when I was a child. Now she is so aware of my needs it is almost as if she is making up for lost time – and she is, in a most profound way. I am deeply touched.

A gargle is to clean out and freshen. It is possible, with a stretch of the imagination, that when I said, 'What you think is what you get', I may have enabled her to refresh her thinking and imagine her feet dancing again.

Mum: *We are together ... in our thinking, Margaret.*
Me: *Yes, Mum, we are and it is truly wonderful.*

'Parallel thoughts', 'together in our thinking' – this sense of togetherness is very strong for her right now and very special for me, too. It sometimes seems that we are reflecting each other's thoughts to one another. Are we actually influencing each other's thoughts, I wonder?

I am struck by how she just knows. I can relate to her because I have learned about the spiritual dimension but her sensitivity, awareness and wisdom come from a very deep level of knowing.

Saturday 7 February 2004

Mum is in her room, sitting in her chair. I am massaging her hands and feet, playing music and chatting. There is no particularly insightful information.

Sunday 8 February 2004

Everything is much the same as yesterday. There is no new information but lots of appreciation for my attention and healing touches.

Monday 9 February 2004

The same again, lots of expressions of appreciation.

Mum: *Something I wanted to tell you, I can't remember. Something happened to my brain. Tele-vision has been marvellous. A huge number of things to think about – can't remember.*

Recalling what she told me three months ago about an injection in her brain, I wonder if this is still happening.

And I guessed correctly – it seems her inner 'tele-vision' is her portal to the Other World. She is accessing the Other World frequently these days, gaining information that she is clearly enjoying.

I am aware that although she can think clearly, she can't always remember.

I decide to ask her one of the big questions.

Me: *What is really important, Mum?*
Mum: *The soul.*

Now she is talking about the soul as if she really knows it, unlike at the beginning of our journey when she asked me, 'Do I have a soul?' I believe that being open to her Other World over the last six months has enabled her to find the other lost parts of herself and reconnect with her soul again.

Tuesday 10 February 2004

Mum is in her room, sitting in a chair and looking very snug. She asks me if we can watch TV, something she has never done before. I switch on the TV and to my amazement a programme is just starting on the subject of reincarnation. She and I watch it together with great interest. The coincidence of the timing of her unusual request with this subject matter is remarkable: another example of her highly intuitive powers. When this programme

87

ends, rather than continuing to watch, she asks to have the TV switched off. So she tuned in for a purpose.

Wednesday 11 February 2004

It is a nice day so in the afternoon I decide to take Mum out in the car, to give her a change of scene. Going out is desirable but also quite a performance for someone with Mum's level of disability, and it is not surprising that after a few attempts many people give up on excursions away from the care facilities.

First, there is the struggle of trying to get her very stiff arms into the sleeves of her oversized coat without hurting her. Then, the frequent problem of finding a wheelchair that has both feet; the feet are detachable and one always seems to be missing. (Where they disappear to remains a complete mystery!) Then there is the complication of finding a member of staff who is free to unlock the door for us, at the same time stopping other residents from escaping. Once we are safely free, I then require assistance from a member of staff to help me to lift Mum from the wheelchair into the car, a backbreaking job despite her petite frame and feather-light weight. And finally, once she is safely ensconced in the car, the wheelchair needs to be returned to the home. It can take at least half an hour just to get to the point of being ready to leave. And we must do this all again in reverse when we return.

At last we make our way to the first of our favourite spots. I park the car in a prime viewing point overlooking the sea and open the windows to let the fresh air swirl around us. It is welcome and bracing. We sit in silence and behold the ocean before us. In the distance the mountain peaks of the Isle of Arran are faintly silhouetted against the sky, like a Japanese painting. The weak winter sun is glinting off the water. Below us, the sea is breaking over the rocks, while giant seagulls glide in the wind and swoop down into the water to catch their food. We appreciate the beauty and wonder of this world.

After a while we turn away from the sea and head a mile or so inland to the second of our favourite places in nature.

small chunks of information sequentially. I wonder where her instructions to do this have come from. Is it through her inner knowing or has she received a message to do this?

Mum: *Like bookends holding things together so that Margaret won't have much to do.*

Again she is thinking of Margaret and trying to protect me. I am deeply touched. It sounds as if she is trying to hold things together and keep them in place for my sake.

Mum: *It would be awful not to be able to walk. It can happen.*

She keeps moving her legs to keep them working while seated in her chair. On a good day she can still walk a very short distance with assistance and is eager to do so. I am pleased to hear her next remark, made despite her physical limitations.

Mum: *I am at peace. I have no worries and no fear.*

This is a state of surrender. I am relieved she is at peace as she is still very aware of everything around her. Before she had Alzheimer's, she could never have made these two statements as she was in a constant state of anxiety.

Wednesday 7 April 2004

Paul is here again and he and I make a brief visit to Mum, whom we find sitting comfortably in her room.

Paul: *Hello Granny! It's nice to see you.*
Mum: *Hello Paul.*
Me: *Hello Mum. How are you?*
Mum: *Average.*
      Here we are. It's complete. I have no worries.
Paul: *That's good Granny.*

93

I think having her daughter and her grandson with her is helping her to feel complete. I notice again how inhibited I feel when Paul is around and how this affects the way I interact with Mum. We all remain very much in this world. I wouldn't think of dancing around the room or venturing into discussions about the Other World.

Afterwards, I have a brief moment of self-doubt and ask myself: 'Is what is happening with Mum real? Am I making all this up?' I have my notes and tapes so the evidence is all there. But this moment of doubt demonstrates the very delicate nature of our Other World connection and the necessity for creating a sacred space in order for it to manifest.

Friday 9 April 2004

It would have been my late sister's birthday today. I mention it to Mum and we remember her together. Dad and I don't talk about it. He has moved on and Fiona seems to have been forgotten.

Saturday 10 April 2004

Mum is in her room, looking quite bright.

Mum: *These are precious moments.*
       I hope I will be able to speak to you.
Me: *You are speaking to me now.*
Mum: *That is past, I mean in the future.*

She is absolutely correct and still able to think in linear time (left-hemisphere brain activity). So these statements are made from this world rather than the Other World. She is also aware of the progressive nature of Alzheimer's disease and the possibility that she may not be able to walk or speak at some time in the future. It has been on my mind, too, and I truly hope it won't come to that. Has she read my mind? After having had such rich and meaningful communication, it would be very sad for both of us if we could no longer converse.

Thursday 22 April 2004

I have been in London but have had to return to Scotland unexpectedly to deal with an emergency with Dad, so it is less than two weeks since I have seen Mum. After a busy day I visit her. She is in her room and in good spirits. It is clear she is having thoughts and is eager to share them with me but a second later she can't remember what they were.

Me: *Hello Mum. It's lovely to see you looking so bright. How are you feeling?*
Mum: *Fine.*
       I had an operation. I am getting better. I feel good. William has had an operation, too.

Well, this is interesting news! I wonder what change I will see in Dad. I have an idea what this might be about.

Me: *Your operation – anywhere in particular?*
Mum: *In my head.*
Me: *Anywhere in particular in your head?*
Mum: *Everywhere.*
Me: *How did you do that?*
Mum: *I asked them. It's that simple.*

I am reminded of this line from Matthew 7:7, 'Ask and it shall be given you: seek and ye shall find.'
       I am lying on the bed hugging her. I have something important to tell her.

Me: *I am sorry to have to tell you this, Mum, but Dad has had a fall. He has fractured his pelvis and is in hospital.*
Mum: *Oh dear, I am sorry to hear that.*

This kind of fracture is extremely painful and difficult for someone of Dad's age. I wonder if there might be a link between the operation Mum said he'd had and his fall. He didn't have a physical operation as such, but maybe the shock and the pain rendered him vulnerable and as a result opened him to the kind of 'operation' Mum described having.

I am busy dealing with Dad in hospital and in crisis. This is putting extra stress on me both emotionally and physically. The hospital is about 15 miles away so travelling to visit him several times a day, in addition to seeing Mum, is very demanding.

Saturday 24 April 2004

Mum is in her room and we are talking.

Mum: *Emily, she needs to grow up.*

Emily is thirty. The difficulties she experienced in the womb, at birth and in childhood undoubtedly affected her. But no one would know this from looking at her or talking to her now. She is indeed young for her years but she is absolutely lovely and things are definitely starting to change.

Mum: *You have a lovely face.*
Me: *Thank you, Mum.*

Friday 7 May 2004

Evening. Mum is sitting up in bed, looking good.

Me: *Hello Mum. It's lovely to see you. How are you?*
Mum: *Fine.*

I haven't seen Mum all week. I have been laid up with flu, having been very overstretched by Dad's crisis. She looks radiant and says nothing is on her mind. Then out of the blue she lifts one hand very slowly and, looking at it thoughtfully, says:

Mum: *I'm getting this hand ready to say goodbye. It must be.*

This is such a symbolic and moving gesture that tears start to well up in me. I have missed my intimate times with her in the wake of Dad's fall and wonder if she has, too.

Mum: *I've done well to preserve my body and keep it in good working order.*
Me: *Yes you certainly have, Mum.*
Mum: *William will be all right. I've passed on ...*
Me: *What have you passed on Mum?*
No reply.

So she is continuing to help Dad and I wonder what she has passed on to him. She could be seeing herself in a future state, after 'passing on' from this life, but this is not the phraseology she would normally use. I leave the care home in floods of tears with the image of her touching gesture in my heart. The duty nurse is very caring toward me. The staff are completely unaware of the extraordinary experiences Mum and I are having. Mum to them is a graceful old lady whom they love, and I am seen as a deeply caring daughter who visits her frequently.

Sunday 23 May 2004

I haven't seen Mum for a couple of weeks. She is in the residents' lounge and I take her down to her room.

Me: *Hello Mum. It's lovely to see you. How are you feeling?*
Mum: *Average.*
       The new tele-vision programme – I don't want it. I'm not happy with it.

Oh dear, this is not good news. How did this happen when she seemed to be so positive in this realm and have everything under control? Did she just make a poor choice of programme? Or might she still have some lessons to learn? Could this be the third initiation on her spiritual journey, the one relating to the mental level of the human energy field, through which she will gain mastery over her thoughts?

Me: *What are you not happy with Mum?*
No reply.

When she doesn't reply it suggests it is something coming from the Other World. I don't believe she is withholding anything from me. Maybe she just knows, but the information doesn't come in the form of words. Whatever the reason for her silence, I respect her position and don't push her.

Thursday 10 June 2004

Mum is in her room, sitting in a chair. Her voice is very weak but her eyes are bright and searching.

Me: *Hello Mum. How are you?*
Mum: *Fine.*

I decide to take her out in the car to our special places by the sea and in the woods. Sitting in the car, looking out at the sea, I ask her what she is thinking.

Mum: *I see shapes.*
She repeats this at different times.
Me: *Show me the shapes you are seeing.*

Very slowly she lifts her stiff arms, nearly above her head, and without speaking starts moving them and her body in a swaying motion, mirroring the undulating movement of the sea before us. This is a truly magic moment and an exquisite expression of the dancer that lives on in her despite her physical limitations. This was and still is Mum – movement is the language of her soul. It is through this kind of creative expression that she finds her freedom and her spirit. Such unity between body and spirit is captured by WB Yeats in his poem 'Among School Children' that ends:

> O body swayed to music, O brightening glance,
> How can we know the dancer from the dance?

Friday 11 June 2004

Mum is in her room.

Mum: *I'm finding my spirit and it feels good.*

I am holding her hand, imagining both our crown chakras open.

Mum: *You are ... a private part where only I can feel.*

The crown chakra is located at the top of the head and is one of seven main chakras or energy centres in the body. It has the fastest vibration and highest frequency, and is the centre that connects us most directly with Spirit. I have often sent Mum healing energy, which she really appreciates, but this is the first time I have focused on the crown centre specifically. I am surprised by her comment about a 'private part' and can only imagine that she is instructing me not to go there because, being closer to Spirit than I am, her crown chakra is functioning at a higher frequency than mine and so our frequencies are not aligned.

Mum: *You have lovely hands, a lovely face. I love you so much, Margaret.*

This is unconditional and from the heart, and it opens my heart.

Me: *I love you too, Mum. You are wonderful. Know that you are.*

Saturday 12 June 2004

It is a lovely summer's day and we are heading off to a favourite little tearoom in town that we have been going to for years. As I push the wheelchair along the pavement toward the promenade, I catch the familiar smell of the sand, a smell that I have only ever associated with this part of the beach and which I can almost taste. It transports me right back to my childhood and the times I spent with my sister and cousins playing on the beach and in the sand dunes and splashing around in the sea. Not so long ago I was doing the same thing with my little son and niece. My parents were younger and fitter then and would come to join us – such happy memories.

The wheelchair squeaks and bumps along the uneven surface of the promenade. In places we are sheltered from the sea breeze by the sand dunes. As we slowly trundle along we engage with lots of friendly faces: little children in pushchairs reaching out, bigger children on and off their bikes, and elderly people walking their little dogs. Then we look along the beach and out to sea. In a few weeks' time, when the summer holidays start, it will be very busy with day-trippers from Glasgow down to enjoy a day at the sea.

After a leisurely thirty-minute stroll we arrive at the tearoom, one that is wheelchair-friendly. We have tea and freshly baked fruit scones with butter. Mum says it's lovely. However, this time she has some difficulty eating and drinking and I have to help her.

Mum: *I feel stupid. I'm so old.*

I feel upset that I have put her in this situation. She feels self-conscious and I realize this is probably the last time we will venture into a public place of this kind. What does her discomfort say about our society and how it views the old? The question makes me feel incredibly sad.

I am returning to London tomorrow and will be back again soon for Mum's birthday.

Tuesday 22 June 2004

I have been here for a couple of days and today is Mum's eighty-ninth birthday. I give her a bunch of sweet peas, her favourite flower, and she enjoys their delicate fragrance and beautiful colours. Unfortunately, Mum is very poorly. She has a rattling cough and is on antibiotics again.

Me: *Hello Mum. How are you today? That sounds like a nasty cough. How are you feeling?*
Mum: *Fair.*
      It will happen some day, Margaret. I love you. You have a lovely face.
Me: *I love you too, Mum. I'm sorry you are not so well.*
Mum: *I'm trying to separate my bones.*

She is aware of how frail she is and constantly reminds me.

I love her poetic way of saying things. Her mobility is worsening, as happens with Alzheimer's disease, and as a result she has become very stiff. Having been a physical education teacher and a dancer she has a great awareness of her physical body and the need to stretch her skeletal frame.

In the afternoon I bring her round to the house for a birthday tea. Dad, Emily and a few close friends are here and she gets lots of cards and good wishes.

Wednesday 23 June 2004

Morning. Mum is in her room.

Mum: *I'm me and you're you.*

I don't know why she is saying this. Am I being too intrusive? I wasn't consciously doing anything but maybe my energy is too strong and I need to tune in and be more sensitive. I respect that Mum knows so I am happy to follow her guidance.

Evening. Mum's cough is lifting a little. We are talking. She is rubbing her nose and her brow in an up-and-down movement.

Mum: *Keeps my brain working.*

This repetitive movement may indeed be activating her brain and also her third eye, the invisible eye with beyond ordinary perception. Mum has frequently reported information that seems to have come to her through this channel; for example, her inner tele-vision.

Anatomically, the two hemispheres of the brain meet at the front of the head along a vertical central line so it is possible that rubbing here may stimulate the brain.

Thursday 24 June 2004

Morning.

Mum: *I want to move but I don't know where I want to move to. The Old Testament will do. I am old. You are lovely.*

I understand her use of the word 'move' to mean moving on from this life. A testament can be a covenant between God and man. Her words suggest she is thinking about dying. I wish I could help her but I can't.

Afternoon. It is a lovely day so I bring Mum round to our house for tea. I find it hard work pushing the wheelchair over the chippings in the parking area outside our house. On the left a mass of pink roses climbs the party wall separating our house and the care home.

This has been my parents' home for over twenty years. Like many of the houses in the area it was built in the architectural style of Charles Rennie Mackintosh around the turn of the twentieth century. Today its pristine white roughcast walls and red clay-tiled roof stand out against the blue sky. Seagulls squawk from the rooftop and a southwesterly breeze carries the smell of the sea, only a stone's throw away. The south-facing garden is sunny and bright. Honeysuckle climbs up the front wall, while roses and neatly planted lobelia, allium and petunia provide a colourful border. The lawn is like a putting green; there isn't a weed in sight.

Mum, Dad and I have tea in the garden and it seems as if nothing has changed. Dad gets impatient, goes inside and comes out again. I potter around the garden. Mum sits in her wheelchair looking frail but content. I am conscious of the fact that I am returning to London tomorrow and feel sad. I always tell Mum before I go, to prepare her.

Me: *I find it so hard going away and leaving you, Mum.*
Mum: *You look beautiful with tears, Margaret.*

We have a very honest exchange. On several occasions I close my eyes and feel our energies connecting and radiating.

Mum: *That's nice.*

She always notices when I connect energetically with her, even when I am not saying anything or in physical contact. I know that as her condition deteriorates this is something I can continue to do silently at any time, and I take great comfort from knowing this.

Monday 12 July 2004

I am seeing Mum again after being away for a few weeks. She is in her room, sitting up in bed. Her voice is weak and she is closing her eyes but is still awake.

Me: *Hello Mum. How are you? You look a little sleepy.*
Mum: *I am feeling average.*
          I'm strong, I keep going.
Me: *What do you think keeps you going?*
Mum: *Breathing.*

Of course we need to breathe to stay alive, but Mum is placing special emphasis on the healing qualities of the breath.

Mum: *I think of William. He needs help. He isn't a good communicator.*

She is right in one sense. Although Dad is the life and soul of the golfing fraternity and never short of a joke, he does not know how to communicate with her. When I tried to talk to him sensitively about this he defended himself immediately by saying, 'I told her that her hair looked nice.' Venus and Mars!

Mum: *These are precious moments. Lovely moments. Your eyes are so bright. Your teeth are lovely. When you smile you have a lovely face.*
Me: *Thank you, Mum. You bring out the best in me.*

Tuesday 13 July 2004

Mum looks brighter.

Mum: *I love you very much. We all have to go sometime. I can read your eyes.*

I take a moment to contemplate this. She keeps reminding me that she is going to go and, although I know it, I still find it hard to think about her not being here, about us not having these precious moments together. However, I believe she has the wisdom to go when the time is right so I am not holding her back.

It is interesting to reflect on how long she has been talking about going, nearly a year now, and she is still here. I wonder if she is finding our journey stimulating with all its revelations and whether this is motivating her to continue.

When Mum looks at me with her unfaltering gaze, I sometimes find it difficult to stay connected because I feel utterly transparent. I need to work on this. What don't I want her to see? What do I not want to see in myself?

Sunday 1 August 2004

I am here for Dad's ninety-third birthday; to look at him, you would never believe he is this age. My niece has come down from Glasgow and some family friends have joined us for a birthday tea. Mum is fine but quiet as usual. Dad is in great form. He loves social occasions like this and being the centre of attention.

Thursday 5 August 2004

I have been here for nearly a week and have been visiting regularly but have nothing in particular to report.

Me: *Hello Mum. How are you today? How are you feeling?*
Mum: *Fine.*
         I'm hearing words and saying them backward in my head.
Me: *What words are you hearing?*
No reply.

What words? What is the purpose of this exercise? Could she be experiencing a little-known phenomenon called 'reverse speech'? In normal speech we hear what is being said at a conscious level. However, when the same message is recorded and played back in reverse, a different but still meaningful message is audible. It is believed that this message comes from the unconscious so is a statement of truth.

Friday 6 August 2004

Mum is in bed and is free-associating – the words she is saying seem to be coming uncensored from her unconscious mind. Then she says:

Mum: *I am progressing in my own time. I want to do it properly.*

She is describing dying as a process, one that involves a degree of self-determination. True to form she wants to do it properly.

Mum: *Margaret and Fiona, how are they?*

Again she refers to me in the third person and I wonder why. Fiona is dead and she is talking about Fiona and me as if we are together. I'm sure we are in her mind, but are we together in the Other World, too? This is intriguing and mystifying and I would love to know more.

Mum: *The book, she read the book.*
Me: *What book, Mum? Who read the book?*
No reply.

Who is 'she'? Might it be Fiona? 'What book?' I ask her, but as this message is coming from the other side, as usual Mum is silent. Could she possibly be referring to the Book of Life, the Akashic Records? This is the infallible collection of all the knowledge of the cosmos said to exist in the Other World. Might Mum have accessed these records?

Mum: *Fiona laid down the law.*
      I want to know Margaret is settled in her home and she isn't.

It sounds as if it was indeed Fiona who read the book. What law is Mum referring to? The Akashic Records are said to contain the universal laws.

It is true that I am not settled. I don't know to what extent this is due to living in two places.

Mum: *Your teeth are so white and regular. You are a lovely girl. What are you thinking?*
Me: *I am thinking of 'being' and angels.*
Mum: *I know the angels and communicate with them.*
Me: *How lovely, Mum. That doesn't surprise me.*

Monday 9 August 2004

Mum: *I need to keep active or I will die. I don't want to die yet.*

Mum is fretting and shaking as she says this, so I hold her gently but firmly. She is right about needing to keep active and is trying so hard to do this. In an attempt to divert her attention and relieve her distress, I show her photos that I have brought in on my laptop to show her.

Mum: *I can't do things now.*

The presence of my laptop and technology with which she is not familiar may have prompted this remark, so I make a mental note to be more sensitive to this in future and introduce new things in a non-threatening way. I know that seeing the photos would do her good.

Me: *But you can be rather than do.* Being *is more important.*

The title of the most famous book by the spiritual teacher Ram Dass is *Be Here Now*. In it, he says that *being* rather than giving and receiving is the most important aspect of love.

Mum: *Margaret has a wonderful future. Margaret has a copy.*
That's good.
Me: *Thank you, Mum. You have made me curious now.*

I imagine that when she is talking to Margaret, she is talking
to my energy body, which she is seeing in her mind's eye. But
if Margaret's energy body has a copy, where is it? I wonder
if it resides somewhere in the spiritual planes. The mystery
of the nature and location of me, Margaret and Margaret's
copy deepens.

The precise meaning of what Mum is saying is not always
clear to me.

Mum: *You'll enjoy the course on chemicals. I found there was*
one piece, file missing. I've done it now, filled it in.

This sounds as if she may have accessed information about body
chemistry and, finding a deficiency, taken corrective action.
Considering her previous comment about 'an injection in my
brain', she may be talking about a process on a different plane.

Mum: *I've been doing exercises.*
Me: *What exercises?*
Mum: *Numbers, I can't remember.*

I wonder if she is referring to numerology – the system of
esoteric healing based on numbers.

Mum: *You have a lovely face, Margaret.*
Me: *You're always searching for the truth, Mum.*
Mum: *Yes, that's exactly right.*

Mum looks happy that I have recognized this important
aspect of her or, more accurately, of her soul. She finds this
deeply affirming.

Tuesday 10 August 2004

Mum is bright and eager to talk.

Mum: *I've been working on my plan to leave. I've done two things on the list. I want everything to be worked out. I don't know who is going to keep Margaret company. Margaret is looking after her health.*
Emily has learned a lot. She showed me her study last night.

I am very touched that she is continuing to think about 'Margaret's' needs and my potential loneliness once she has gone. Having chosen to make my parents the priority in my life, I don't have the time and energy just now to nourish and sustain the relationship I am in and she seems to be aware of this. I don't know what the future will hold for me when she and Dad have gone.

I have noticed that Emily is progressing, as Mum says. It seems that they are communicating but on a level that Emily, as far as I know, is not consciously aware of. Could it be through dreams, I wonder?

I am holding Mum's feet and gently massaging them.

Mum: *What you are doing has made me very relaxed.*
Margaret will meet the new assistant. She has shoulder-length red curly hair.

I haven't met any new assistant in the care home, but maybe Margaret has a new guide in Mum's Other World.

Wednesday 11 August 2004

Mum is bright and very lucid.

Mum: *Margaret, make sure you have all the information to take to the doctor person.*

I don't know what she is referring to. It could relate to my recent request to her doctor for approval to give Mum vitamin supplements that have been found to help people with Alzheimer's. Or perhaps it is something to do with my own health.

Mum: *There's something wrong with the way Margaret is being brought up. She will put it right. She needs to find out how to govern her own output, work on her own systems. We'll both do that. I'm making a speech.*

'There's something wrong with the way Margaret is being brought up.' Does this relate to now or is Mum recalling my childhood as if it is happening now? Whatever the timing, what she is saying is true. 'Margaret' and I are putting all that right by engaging in this profoundly healing journey with her.

Here are clear instructions for Margaret – for me. Margaret and I have a tendency to give out more than we take in and get overstretched as a result. We need to pay attention to this and make changes.

Mum: *All these brain levels – they're not doing anything much. I want everything to be worked out.*

It is undoubtedly true that, as a result of having Alzheimer's, many of Mum's 'brain levels' are not doing much. But she is still thinking with great clarity a lot of the time, so where is her thinking taking place? It seems to me that her brain is having problems remembering what she knows. As all spiritual teachers tell us, including contemporary teachers like Eckhart Tolle, it is not the brain that is important, but the mind.

Mum: *The new book I have is useful.*
Me: *What new book Mum?*
No reply.

Her comments suggest that she is continuing to learn, possibly from the Book of Life or Akashic Records to which I referred a few days ago.

———————————

I know I was around during September and October and that I saw Mum, but I don't have any record of our time together. This surprises me, but I may just not have had the energy to keep up my journal as I was preoccupied with caring for Dad who was suffering one crisis after another in rapid succession.

———————————

Tuesday 16 November 2004

Mum is in her room. I haven't seen her for a few weeks. She is looking a little flat.

Me: *Hello Mum. It's lovely to see you again. How are you? How are you feeling?*
Mum: *Average. I'm bored.*

She said this twice today and I wonder if the lack of stimulation from me, as a consequence of my attention being on Dad, has led to this feeling. If this is so, it confirms my thought that my usual pattern of intensive visiting periods, during which I give her my undivided attention, is better than the more routine visits I have been making recently.

Mum: *Margaret is careless sometimes but I don't mind a bit.*

Oops! I am unaware exactly what I have been careless about, but Mum doesn't mind, so it's OK. Perhaps she did experience my lessened attention as careless.

Mum: *You have lovely teeth, lovely eyes, a lovely face ...*

Wednesday 17 November 2004

Mum is in her room.

Mum: *I'm looking in my diary, when I'm leaving. Margaret and I can be in the house together. We can talk on the phone. I don't want any jealousy. I want to go to southern Ireland.*

I am pleased and relieved to know that Mum and I will be together when she leaves.

Jealousy is an unexpected word for her to introduce and I have no idea what she is referring to. She may have drifted into childhood memories, as she goes on to talk about Ireland, where her mother came from and where, as a child, she visited her cousins with her siblings.

Me: *We can go together.*

I am giving her some healing energy and offer to take her on a guided visualization.

Mum: *That's lovely.*

She always responds when I tune in and feel our energies flowing together.

Then, out of the blue:

Mum: *Do you prefer brown or blue eyes?*
Me: *Brown.*
Mum: *You have a choice.*

She says this with such certainty. This is the voice of a mystic. Is she talking about a future incarnation?

Mum: *The letters from Fiona or Margaret.*
Me: *What letters?*
No reply.

112

I am deeply curious about these letters and wonder what they contain. As she didn't reply to my question I presume that they are from the Other World.

She continues to talk about Fiona and Margaret together.

I am here, but Fiona is in the Other World. So where is Margaret?

Thursday 18 November 2004

When I visited Mum in the morning she was fine but this evening she is not in a good state.

Mum: *I don't know what's wrong. I don't feel right. I'm still here.*
I'm looking for my diaries.

She is clearly distressed. It is as if she is experiencing being here and, at the same time, not being here. I wonder if her diaries give her a sense of the time-related reality that she is losing.

In the past she kept diaries in which she recorded her thoughts and feelings. Recently I came across one and it made very sad reading. Although she managed her life much better after she returned to teaching, her diaries revealed that she continued to suffer from depression and anxiety. I wasn't fully aware of this at the time. All I can do now is to be present with her, hold her lovingly and reassure her.

Friday 19 November 2004

Mum: *Your thoughts will carry you through. There is always a way round.*

Thankfully, she seems to have pulled through yesterday's mini-crisis.

PROCLAMATION

'Everything, my ideas, thoughts, are from ...'
Pat

Thursday 9 December 2004

I have just arrived back from London and Mum is in bed. She opens her eyes and is surprised to see me. There is pure love shining from her. It is palpable and beautiful.

Me: *Hello Mum. I love you.*
She smiles.
Mum: *I'm doing well. I'm looking and waiting. Both of you have helped me.*

I am waiting, too. 'They also serve who only stand and wait' – as John Milton wrote in 'On His Blindness'.

Is Mum talking about Fiona and Margaret, Fiona and me or Margaret and me?

Mum: *Everything, my ideas, thoughts, are from Fiona. She's done it.*

What? I can't believe I am hearing this. I said I was going to keep an open mind but, well, this is a real test. So far everything Mum has said I have felt intuitively to be true, so I have no reason not to believe her now. But this is a stretch, a huge leap of faith. It seems that the black sheep of the family is now its shining light and saviour.

I am struggling to accept that the presence in the Other World guiding my mother, and the fount of all this wisdom that I have been noting down, could be my so troubled younger sister.

An alcoholic for twenty-five years, she caused a lot of pain for herself and our family and didn't show any interest in spiritual matters. But now, having taken on board what Mum has told me, I am starting to wonder if my sister's purpose in this life might not have been to go first and prepare the way for Mum.

I am remembering now that before Fiona died I had a dream in which she was giving me a special gift. Given the circumstances at the time I couldn't for the life of me think what it might be. I was angry with her for the trail of destruction she was leaving. Now it appears the meaning of that dream might just have been revealed to me.

So it seems that Fiona is helping my mum, my dad, her daughter Emily and me. How wonderful. How unimaginable at the time of her death.

I need to stop and take in the magnitude of this revelation and feel it, really feel it.

As I said, I have wondered if Mum has been reading my mind and speaking my thoughts back to me. But this way of looking at Fiona has never entered my consciousness before. So on this occasion at least I can dismiss that idea.

Mum: *I know my thoughts are clear. I'm confused when I can't remember.*

Mum is making an important distinction between thoughts and memory. She is also telling me that what she has just said is clear – in other words, I am to believe her. How well she communicates what she wants me to know.

Mum: *You are lovely, every part of you. You are loving, Margaret.*
You are a good mother. You helped me.

This is the first time Mum has spoken of me being *her mother* and it does feel as if our roles are now reversed. I am glad she feels this way. As her daughter, having healed my past, I can give her the unconditional love a mother gives her child. Also, with the mind of a therapist, I am able to help her to process and heal the traumas of her life. Of course, this is also healing for my own life.

It is time for me to do what mothers do – tell stories. So, with her sitting up in bed comfortably, I start to reminisce with her and take her on a journey into our past, talking about where we lived when I was growing up, the house, the garden and lots of positive things associated with that time.

Mum: *It seemed awful at the time but it has all come right.*
Me: *Yes it has, Mum, and like you I'm deeply grateful.*

I imagine that our journey into the past, although I focused on the positive things, has stimulated some emotional memories, the 'it' referring to our lives and our relationship. I am so glad she feels it has come right. I need to stop and really take this in. It is a huge achievement and deeply healing for both of us.

Mum: *I'm moving my legs so that I will be able to walk tomorrow.*
     You have to keep doing that. Tomorrow, another nothing
     day. You are clever. You have a good brain.

She is making an astute observation along the lines of 'use it or lose it' and is sounding so disempowered. It must be a struggle and depressing to know that you are losing the battle physically and mentally. In contrast I may seem very fit and able. My heart goes out to her. Her comment 'another nothing day' is uncharacteristic and I wonder if she may once again be depressed. I need to pay attention to this.

Mum: *Margaret needs to dance.*

She is so right, I do, and this is a reminder that I need to get out and have some fun. The kind of dancing I love is different from hers, but when I dance for her I try to express myself to the music in the way she would have done and, despite the clumsiness of my attempts, she loves it.

Mum: *When I look back on my life I ask, 'What was it about? What did I do?'*

These questions are especially pertinent in Mum's case as she had such a difficult life. I want to remind her of the positive things so we talk about her life, its meaning and what she contributed. We talk about the joy she brought to her parents, her brother and her sister. About the gift of life she gave to Fiona and me. The vitality she brought to our home when she was well. How, when we were unwell as children, she looked after us with such loving care. The beautiful smocked dresses she made for us. The delicious cakes she baked.

We talked about the richness of experience she brought to the children she taught. The part she played in introducing dance and creative movement into Scottish schools. The valuable work she did in her pastoral role, supporting and empowering young women.

We talked about how she provided a loving home for Emily and brought her up to be a fine young woman. Her love of the arts: her creativity, her musical talent and her ability to see and enjoy movement in everything around her. Her special friendships and her love of cats.

We talked about the wisdom and insight she has given me on this journey, which are such a wonderful gift. About how she has learned to endure and how she has finally found peace and resolution.

So, in the remembering, together we validate all the positive things in her past. This life review has given us time to appreciate her life and I am seeing her in a positive, shining light, as she is now.

Christmas 2004

Another Christmas, another year, and despite more rehearsals and near misses Mum, thankfully, is still here with us. Like last year, she spends some of the time in the care home participating in the festivities there and some with the family in our house. As usual, she is quiet and reflective in the midst of all the people and talk. My cousin and his wife have joined us, and Dad, who loves social occasions, is on top form.

During the holidays, when Paul and Emily are around, I step back and let them visit their granny.

Sunday 26 December 2004

I make a brief visit just to say hello.

Me: *Hello Mum. You're looking well. How are you feeling?*
Mum: *Fine.*
     [Emphatically] *Love never dies.*

What a wonderful message for us all.

Monday 27 December 2004

Mum: *I need to be independent. I dream, it's good. Things I remember from the past – not so good.*

So her past still seems to haunt her. I spend some time with her and we identify these difficult past events, revisiting them, discovering new ways of looking at them and finding reconciliation. I understand her need for redemption in this critical phase before she dies. Akin to the last rites, this is an opportunity for her to express in words and feelings what she wants to let go of before shuffling off her mortal coil. I am Mum's witness – this is my mission. Following this talk we have a quiet time together.

Wednesday 29 December 2004

Mum: *You have a loving face. Your brown eyes are so bright.*

I am now resting my head next to hers and our cheeks are touching.

Mum: *We've never done this before. It's lovely.*

She clearly enjoys this physical contact. Now I know we will be able to connect in this way in the future, when her ability to speak becomes more limited.

2005

Thursday 3 February 2005

It has been a few weeks since my last visit. I arrive to find Mum sitting in the lounge in the care home, looking very distressed. She looks as if she has Bell's palsy: her mouth is distorted and one side of her face is bruised. She is staring vacantly into space. On enquiring I find out that she has been to the dentist who, with the best of intentions, tried to do as much as he could in one visit. Clearly, it was too much. My poor Mum has been traumatized by this treatment both physically and mentally.

I imagine the whole process of getting Mum to the dental surgery and then treating her must have been extremely difficult. What should a dentist do when faced with all these complications? But has it taken a year to follow up my request that she see a dentist? Has she had an infection all this time? If this is the case, it shows how easily things can slip through the net when one is not there all the time to follow up.

Me: *Hello Mum. It's lovely to see you. You're not looking your usual self. What has happened?*
Mum: *I'm fair.*
      I don't want to be here. I'm not myself.

In addition to Mum's dental trauma she has a chesty cough. Faced with her deteriorated condition, I am at a loss as to what to do but decide, as I have been away for a few weeks and know she won't have been out, to take her in the car for a change of scene. Fortunately, this has the desired effect.

Evening. Mum is in her room and sounding brighter. I think my visit is helping her.

Friday 4 February 2005

Mum looks flaccid but nevertheless struggles to keep communicating.

I continue to visit over the next few days but have nothing new to report. Then I am off again to my other life in London.

Friday 25 February 2005

After a few weeks I am back with Mum who is in bed dozing and drifting in and out of sleep.

Me: *Hello Mum. It's really lovely to see you. How are you?*
Mum: *Fine.*

She is fixating on my teeth.

Mum: *You have beautiful teeth.*
         When I leave where will I go? I'll be free!
Me: *Mum, you'll go to wherever you want to go to, wherever*
         you imagine, and you'll most definitely be free.
Mum: *Thank you, Margaret. I'll remember that.*
         I've made good use of this year. I've got everything in place,
         done everything. Margaret has been a great help. She is
         good, very good. It's wonderful to have loving parents.

Her review of the past year confirms her progress in preparation for dying. This is despite having said last May that she'd started a programme she didn't like.

She has been talking about me as her mother and now she is talking about Margaret as her mother. So she is experiencing both Margaret and me as her mother. That's nice.

Me: *What are you thinking? I'm asking because I want to know what it's like being you. I want to understand.*

Mum: *My thoughts, they float by and disappear and I can't catch them, remember them. They are lovely, just lovely, wild.*

I am struck by her words and so pleased she is having lovely wild thoughts, even if she can't remember them to tell me. This sounds like she is finding her spirit. How wonderful!

Her description brings to mind one of her most loved songs, 'The Windmills of Your Mind' sung by Noel Harrison. The poetic lyrics of this song express for me the freedom of the Alzheimer's mind.

Mum's eyes are focused behind me on my left and she is attempting to move but can't, save for stretching out her hand as if intent on reaching something.

Me: *What are you seeing, Mum?*
Mum: *There's something there.*
Me: *What?*

She can't describe it.

Mum: *That was lovely, absolutely lovely.*
    [After a pause] *Margaret has dreams.*

She is clairvoyant! I have just had a dream about her.

Me: *Yes, Mum, and you were in my dreams. I dreamed that I was teaching and you came along in the lunch break and*

*joined my students and me. Then a Jeep Cherokee people
carrier came to collect you.*

Mum: *The spirit world is wonderful.*

Dreaming is an activity of the mind and when we dream, according to many spiritual and shamanic teachings, a part of us goes to another dimension, to the Other World. It sounds as if Mum, who seems to be a frequent traveller to that Other World, met me there. Perhaps a Native American spirit carried (guided) her there.

I am sending Mum light.

Mum: *I like that.*

I notice that she is moving her head from side to side again.

Me: *What's happening?*
Mum: *I am ... a tune but I don't want to unravel it.*

She has said before that she hears tunes and changes them into words. I wonder if this is what is happening now. Maybe her mind is tuned into a certain frequency and she is enjoying it so much she doesn't want to 'download' it to her brain. Might she be tuned in to the mystical music of the spheres?

Me: *You are perfect, Mum.*

She visibly glows on hearing this.

These are precious moments. I will remember them for ever. Somehow I feel she will, too.

Saturday 26 February 2005

Mum: *I'm getting ready for the next programme. I need to decide
which programme.*

So she has a choice about the programme. After her dislike of the one she had back in May last year, I hope this one, whatever it is, is right for her. It would seem she is choosing to go on living and learning.

REDEMPTION

'I'm remembering all the difficult times, all the people ...'
Pat

Wednesday 23 March 2005

Having travelled up from London, I arrive at the care home in the
afternoon and find Mum in the lounge with the other residents.

Me: *Hello Mum. It's lovely to see you again. How are you?*
Mum: *Fine.*
Me: *I had another dream about you, Mum. I dreamed that you
       showered yourself and got yourself dressed.*
Mum: *That is how I like to think about myself.*
Me: *Feel free! Imagine it now.*

I wonder if my dream was somehow tuning into Mum in the Other
World. Was I seeing how she will be when she finally makes the
transition from this body that is ready to retire into the Other
World? Is she already in that free state in some dimension?

Evening. Mum is in bed.

Mum: *I have a telephone directory and I can talk to anyone
       I want.*
Me: *That's wonderful Mum. Who do you talk to?*
Mum: *Lots of people. I spoke to Fiona. She came once.
       She's fine.
       She doesn't do more than she's meant to do. Dad, he's just
       there. Mum, she's a hoot. I have Margaret and Fiona.
       They are very different.*

124

So she is telling me that an open channel allows her to contact anyone she wants and that she is in communication with deceased family members in the Other World. This is the first time she has spoken explicitly about her mother and father. Her comment about Margaret and Fiona is true: we were, and are, very different. Interestingly, she says, 'I have Margaret and Fiona,' as if Margaret is there, too. So again it seems that Margaret exists in the Other World as well as in this world. Although I have my own glimpses of non-duality from time to time, I still find it amazing to contemplate.

Mum: *Have I been a good mother, Margaret?*

This is a very difficult question. Mum perceives only the truth so I can't lie about anything, including this. She was a good mother when she was well and she is a very good mother now.

Me: *We have had our difficulties in the past but when you were well you were a good mother. Those times are past and we are fine now. Yes Mum, you are a good mother, in fact you are a wonderful mother.*
Mum: *I can't remember.*

This is a relief to me as she had been agitated and perturbed by her memories and I don't want to dwell on these now unless she needs to. It seems we have truly moved on.

Me: *Fine, no need.*
Mum: *You have a lovely face, kind brown eyes. A face full of feelings, well proportioned.*

It is so nice to know that she really sees me, that Mum and I really see each other. How often do we actually see another person?

Mum: *Emily, how is she? Where is she?*

Me: *She's in Glasgow. She's working hard and still dreams about getting into television. She's fine.*

Mum: *I love when you're here. It makes such a difference ... I get confused.*

Me: *Don't worry.*

I am holding her hand.

Me: *I'm here and I just love being with you.*

Friday 25 March 2005

It is 8.30pm and Mum is in bed, looking very comfortable. I am holding her gently.

Mum: *I've had a difficult life since I was young but I've managed. I had a terrible breakdown but I came through it. We did our best for Margaret but she was battered.*

Oh my! Deep, deep sigh. I am stunned by the brutal frankness of her comment about me. Yes, I was battered, not so much physically as emotionally. This recognition of my pain touches a deep and vulnerable part inside me and I am feeling very tearful. It is the first time she or indeed anyone other than a therapist has acknowledged this for me. Where did this lightning bolt come from? I have a feeling of being empty, in a good way, from hearing Mum acknowledge this truth. I had a difficult life but like her I am a survivor and like her I came through it. Now this final journey together is making it all worthwhile.

My thirty years as a therapist, as well as my personal experience, have shown me that the greatest challenges can lead to life's greatest gifts. Margaret and I wouldn't have had it any other way.

Mum: *Was my life worthwhile?*

Me: *Yes, dearest Mummy, of course it was.*

126

Driving along a narrow country lane with neatly trimmed copper beech hedges and ploughed fields on either side, we are engulfed by the smell of the country. This is the landscape of Mum's childhood and brings back many memories for her. As we round a bend we enter the woods and come across another sea – a sea of snowdrops extending as far as the eye can see. We take time to wonder at this magical white carpet that has grown, undisturbed by mankind, over many lifetimes. We pause and take time to wonder at this beautiful canvas created by Mother Nature. Further along, in a clearing in the wood, we stop and watch children in a little playground that nestles naturally in its surroundings. Seeing young ones brings great joy to Mum. Then we are homeward bound and back in time for tea.

This short outing not only reconnects Mum with the outside world and forgotten special places, but also allows us to appreciate the wonder of nature together. She can fill her lungs with much-needed fresh air and so can I. Trips like this break up the monotony of being in the care home; I also notice when we are out and about that her focus is outward rather than inward and our conversations reflect this. So although getting going is an enormous effort, it is always worth it and she is worth it.

Evening. I take Mum down to her room so that we can talk in peace and quiet.

Mum: *You are my comforter, Margaret.*
I need to expand my activities. I don't like just sitting in my chair. It's been a busy day. I can't remember with what.

Although she doesn't recollect our outing this afternoon, it seems on some visceral level to have reminded her of the world out there and her desire to be part of it. It doesn't matter that she doesn't recall what we did a few hours ago; it is what is happening now, in the moment, that matters.

Mum: *You have good dreams.*

It is true, I do have good dreams, and I have always attached great importance to them. It was through my dreams that I had deep insights into my psyche and discovered the hidden truths that led to my healing and enabled me to emerge from my dark night of the soul.

Mum: *I need a peaceful mind.*
You have such loving eyes and face, Margaret. I've never seen such loving eyes.

It is hard to find words to describe such moments and it is somewhat embarrassing to recount them for you here. But when Mum looks at me and I hear her voice offering such heartfelt appreciation, I feel that I am dissolving, melting away.

Thursday 12 February 2004

Today turned out to be much the same as the previous day.

Friday 13 February 2004

Mum is in bed and looks very contented.

Mum: *I'm appreciating all the gratitude in the world. You have such loving eyes, lovely teeth and face.*
Me: *That's lovely Mum. Thank you.*
Mum: *I feel free. William thinks everything can happen like that. I love my family. I am a good mother. To get the change you have to have an operation.*

Again, there are some important thoughts rolling out together in this stream of consciousness: gratitude, freedom, process, love and change.

She said early on in our journey that freedom was important, so I am glad to be told now that she feels free. To be completely free one must be under no illusions about one's being; one must be free from conditioning and have reclaimed one's true self.

I am pleased too that she has overcome her previous concern about being a 'bad person'.

She has reported having 'operations' to remove things from her mind and says she has improved as a result. Although I can't verify the 'operations', I can say that her mind has definitely improved.

Dad has always been impatient. He likes things to happen quickly and to reach his destination. Mum understands that there is a process and appreciates the journey.

Saturday 14 February 2004

Afternoon. Mum is sitting in her chair in her room. A staff nurse is with us, carrying out a mandatory six-monthly review. With a little encouragement Mum becomes actively engaged and starts to answer the questions very confidently. It is lovely to see; it would be so easy to assume she could not cope with such an interview and take over from her. But to our surprise she is doing very well on her own and feeling very empowered by the experience. The nurse and I are amazed.

Sunday 15 February 2004

Morning. Mum is very bright, leaning forward in her chair and looking the best she has done for years.

Evening. Mum is in bed, very tired and sleepy. I notice a strong smell coming from her body and I know something is wrong, possibly another urinary tract infection. It is shocking how quickly things can change – one minute she can be fine and the next she can be dipping into illness and extreme weakness. I stroke her.

Mum: *You are doing me good. Are you not tired going from one house to the other? You have lovely teeth, a lovely face, and lovely brown eyes.*

I am giving her a gentle hug.

Mum: *You are a darling.*
I've done everything. There are guardian angels all
around me.
Me: *Do they bring you comfort?*
Mum: *I don't need comfort.*
Me: *Do they give you support?*
Mum: *Support is the right word.*

Her concern for me is on-going and it is true that the travelling back and forth between Scotland and London, 'going from one house to the other', is demanding, but it is what I am choosing to do.

It is wonderful that she is sensitive to the angelic realm and can articulate her experiences so succinctly.

I alert the nursing staff to the possibility of an infection. They need to take a sample and send it off for testing to ascertain the most effective antibiotic. This takes time and in the meantime Mum's health and vitality can spiral downward very quickly.

Monday 8–Thursday 11 March 2004

I have been away. On my return I notice straightaway that things have changed since my last visit. Previously, Mum had stored up observations to tell me when I arrived, but this time her attention seems more on the inside. She is constantly counting out loud and trying to work out dates.

Me: *Hello Mum. It's lovely to see you. How are you feeling?*
Mum: *Average.*
I'm trying to keep my brain working.

Counting activates the left hemisphere, the part of the brain that specializes in digital-type communication, in dealing with

I affirm all the positive things in her life and tell her they are the most wonderful gifts.

Mum: *I'm remembering all the difficult times, all the people ...*

Previously, she said she couldn't remember her past difficulties, and I have been trying to protect her from them, but true to form she is persisting in her quest for the truth. Her poignant question suggests she is seeking another life review.

I want to help her now so that she will be completely free of any difficulties when she makes her final transition to the Other World. I have already mentioned the importance of redemption at this stage of life.

Me: *Is there anyone you want to talk about? Anything you want to say?*
Mum: [Emphatically] *I love everyone.*
Me: *That's perfect. That is* complete. *There's no need to do anything more.*
Mum: *I've overcome the difficulties and it's all gone now. I'm at peace. I suffered.*
Me: *I know you did, Mum.*
Mum: *No one else knows that.*
Me: *I know, I'm your witness.*
Mum: *She* [referring to herself] *has overcome.*

Her unequivocal proclamation about universal love has produced a powerful energy that has overridden all previous negative thoughts. My affirmation of this, delivered as an embedded command, anchored a new pattern. I am deliberately using NLP terminology here, as I found the techniques particularly useful in such circumstances; by saying 'That is complete', I encouraged Mum to continue along her new positive thought path. Mum's affirmative response to my statement shows the instant change in perception that can come about in such moments of pure, focused intention. She has indeed overcome and moved on. Referring to

127

herself as 'she' indicates that she is either in a dissociated state or speaking from the Other World.

Only after being greatly tested in this world can we gain the kind of knowledge and wisdom that Mum is accessing now.

This is a very intimate and tender time and I feel tears welling up in me again. She suffered, and having dealt with my own suffering, I am now able to be her witness, her one and only witness. This realization is at the heart of our journey together.

Mum: *I've learned to endure.*
        Margaret is always there.

I understand from this exchange that the Margaret she is constantly talking about is permanent and always available to her. I am very happy about this.

Me: *Yes I am, Mum, and you are always with me.*

Moving from the profound to the profane:

Mum: *What age are you? Fifty-one?*
Me: *No, I'm sixty-two.*
Mum: *You have a lovely face. You have beautiful teeth.*

Saturday 26 March 2005

Evening. Mum is in bed and very bright.

Mum: *Emily ...? Breathing is the answer for everyone.*

I think she might be suggesting that Emily would benefit from using the breath therapeutically, and I gather she wants me to pass this on to my niece, which I am more than happy to do. Our dialogue is having a positive ripple effect.

Mum: *The diaries, I must get it right.*
Me: *What diaries?*

Mum: *I don't know where they are.*

Another reference to her lost diaries, perhaps because organizing and planning her life is becoming impossible for Mum. I imagine the frontal cortex of the brain, the part that performs these tasks, is not working well now. I wish I knew how to help.

Me: *Are you ever fed up, Mum?*
Mum: *No, never.*
Me: *Do you ever feel lonely?*
Mum: *No, never. I'm never alone.*
Me: *Who is with you?*
Mum: *I don't know, but there is someone.*

Mum spends a very long time looking at me, at my eyes.

Mum: *The eyes have it. The eyes are the window to the soul. You have beautiful brown eyes, beautiful teeth, beautiful nails.*

She has shifted her attention from my face to my hands. Now she moves back to the on-going enigma:

Mum: *Margaret and you are very different.*
Me: *Can you describe the difference?*
No reply.
Me: *I am Margaret.*
Mum: *Yes. We are very fortunate.*
Me: *Yes we are, Mum.*

I have wondered previously if she refers to Margaret when she is in a dissociated state and I am therefore one step removed. But then she would experience Margaret and me as being the same. Presumably, when she says 'you', she is perceiving me in physical form. What is the nature and form of Margaret? Is she seeing Margaret in her mind? Is she tuning into my aura? Is she seeing a genetic pattern? Is she seeing my essence?

129

I agree that we are very fortunate but I believe it is possible for everyone to have positive experiences like we are having. One just needs to want it enough.

Sunday 27 March 2005

Continuing to explore the enigma:

Me: *Margaret and me?*
Mum: *I don't know, cousins? Then you would have a brother and sister. That would be nice.*

It is not at all clear what she is thinking about and she seems confused. She is using a future tense, so is it possible that she is seeing a future incarnation? Is this some family constellation from the past that she is now seeing in the future?

Thursday 28 April 2005

Mum is in the lounge with the other residents when I arrive.

Me: *Hello Mum. It's lovely to see you. You are looking well. How are you?*
Mum: *Fine thank you, Margaret.*
       I am tidying up. I need to have everything in order.

Evening. She is in bed and makes no further reference to her previous remark.

Friday 29 April 2005

When I visit Mum, I often just talk about people we know and everyday things and she joins in. Today, Mum merely says that she can't remember what she is thinking.

Saturday 30 April 2005

Morning. I am in Mum's room with her. She is having problems remembering. I do a little kinesiology reflex therapy, holding reflexes on her head that stimulate blood flow to the brain, to try to improve her brain function.

Afternoon. I am walking along the promenade with Mum in the wheelchair. She says she doesn't want to go to the tearoom and I feel saddened by this but understand. I imagine that she is remembering the uncomfortable feelings she had the last time we were there, when she couldn't cope and needed help. So her emotional memory is still functioning.

Evening. Mum is in bed, looking bright. I decide to read to her from a book I think she will like: *The Prophet* by Kahlil Gibran.

Mum: *It's deep. It's religious. This is a lovely book. The language is beautiful.*

I am so glad she is able to appreciate this. Suddenly, I have a thought: might she be able to read with me? After searching deep in a drawer beside her bed, I find her reading glasses. They are dirty so I clean them, then put them on for her. I open the book and give it to her. To my utter amazement she reads fluently with comprehension and she doesn't want to stop. She is so pleased at the realization that she can still read and get pleasure from it. This is a magical moment for both of us. I leave her happily reading to herself. The book is small and not too heavy so she can just about manage to hold it.

The staff nurse reports that Mum was bright and still awake at 2am. I am thrilled. How could I not have thought about this possibility before?

Sunday 1 May 2005

Evening. We have more readings from *The Prophet*. She reads enthusiastically, like a thirsty woman finding water unexpectedly. I leave her reading and she calls out happily to me as I leave.

Mum: *Cheerio*!

This is such a positive, upbeat goodbye, it lifts my heart.

Monday 2 May 2005

Evening. Mum is in bed and sleepy. I am lying down with her and hugging her.

Mum: *These are lovely moments.*

We read from *The Prophet* again.

Mum: *This is a lovely book.*

After talking she says to me:

Mum: *William and I have a plan. There are characters. We'll all three be together.*
Me: *Who? You, Dad and me?*
Mum: *Yes.*

This is a wonderful new integration of our family that has in the past been so dysfunctional. It also suggests that she and Dad are communicating at some other level. Is she seeing us as characters in a play? Now, there is an interesting idea. Is she seeing us together in the Other World? And where does my sister Fiona figure in this?

Wednesday 25 May 2005

It is afternoon when I arrive and Mum is in the lounge with other residents.

Me: *Hello Mum. It's lovely to see you again. How are you? How are you feeling?*
Mum: *Fine.*
     Margaret is sorting things out.

Help! She is psychic! I am dealing with some very sensitive financial matters to do with her and Dad and am feeling extremely uncomfortable about it. This is most definitely not something I want to share with her. Dammit. Apparently I am totally transparent. I can't hide anything. Help! My God, what else does she know?

This is the second example of Mum's extrasensory perception.

Evening. Mum is in the lounge again.

Mum: *Margaret is busy with funds and finance. Margaret is a little confused.*

Her reading of me continues despite my desperate wish to block it out. My goodness, nothing gets past her. I haven't mentioned anything financial to her. I feel totally exposed yet know that her remarks are out of her care and concern for me rather than a desire to snoop or interfere.

This is the third time Mum has tuned in to me and given me a spontaneous, unsolicited psychic reading. She has without question developed telepathic powers yet she is totally unaware of them. Some sceptics say that psychics perform so-called supernatural feats by using trickery. Clearly there is no trickery here – Mum is reading my mind without even knowing she is doing it.

133

Thursday 26 May 2005

Morning. Mum is in her room, sitting in her chair and looking bright.

Me: *Hello Mum. It's lovely to see you. How are you?*
Mum: *Fine.*

We talk a little, while I give her a manicure. I then read from *The Prophet*, the last verse of the section on self-knowledge:

> Say not, 'I have found the truth,' but rather, 'I have
>   found a truth.'
> Say not, 'I have found the path of the soul.'
> Say rather, 'I have met the soul walking upon my path.'
> For the soul walks upon all paths.
> The soul walks not upon a line, neither does it grow
>   like a reed.
> The soul unfolds itself, like a lotus of countless petals.

Mum: *Beautiful!*

Afternoon. We go for a wheelchair walk along the promenade. On one side are the sea and sand dunes; on the other, the grassy slopes are covered with fresh young shrubs and wild flowers. We stop and take time to look at the dog roses. Their soft pink flowers and perfume are so delicate and beautiful. After our walk we go back to the house for tea in the garden. Mum is very quiet, as she often is in Dad's company. He doesn't know what to say to her, and she doesn't know what to say to him.

Evening. I find Mum in bed asleep and she wakes up. She doesn't want me to read to her but is happy for me to talk. So I sit down beside her and start talking quietly about something I have mentioned before and imagine that she is already doing: out-of-body or astral travel. This is when a part of us leaves our physical body and goes to another dimension; it's like being in a dream but awake.

Mum: *We can try to do these things.*
Me: *Yes Mum, actually you are already doing them.*
Mum: *My brother* [deceased] *asked me to visit him and I did.*
Me: *There you are, I told you that you were doing it.*
Mum: *I can do more but I don't want to do too much.*
Me: *I agree Mum. You're very wise.*

I love her openness, her spontaneity and what she is experiencing. It is wonderful.

She knows exactly what I am talking about and understands that too much of this could make her feel ungrounded and disorientated.

This is another meeting with a deceased relative but this time she did the visiting. She really is travelling outside her body. Maybe my talking about astral travelling gave her permission to tell me about her experience. I want to encourage her to enjoy the freedom of being out of her body, knowing that she can come back. Having this experience now will make her final transition to the Other World feel natural and effortless.

Mum: *So much love is coming from your face. You have lovely teeth.*
Margaret is very good. Margaret has helped me.
[After a pause] *The night has many nights.*
Me: *What do you mean, Mum?*
Mum: *I can't explain. Lovely thoughts, Margaret. No worries.*

This is so poetic and takes Margaret and me on a journey of the soul to I don't know where ... maybe the upper astral levels where, mysteriously, many nights are said to reside.

I am silently directing my attention to her aura and imagining 'free' and 'light'.

Mum: *Margaret is home and I am home. You are there and between and joining. Our energies are connected.*

Absolutely wonderful! How exquisitely she expresses herself. This is our soul connection. She is feeling or sensing what I am doing and has described it perfectly, calling this non-physical energy state 'home'.

Mum: *These are precious moments. You will cherish them in the future.*

Yes, these are indeed very precious moments, and my eyes fill with tears of gratitude. This is a very special evening. Some negative thoughts had been blocking me and I had asked for help so that I could be more present. Now I am given this most beautiful gift. 'Thank you.'

Friday 27 May 2005

Afternoon. I take Mum down to her room where we can talk together in peace and quiet.

Mum: *I'm finished. My supervision is complete. The library, lots of books, eight books, I'm counting, one, two, three, four and four more. It will take time but I don't mind.*

She can still count and has a concept of linear time, which means that the left hemisphere of her brain, the side that specializes in processing sequential information, is still working.

So the supervision phase is over and she now has study to do. I try to find out more about the library and the eight books but she can't tell me. In August last year she made a reference to someone reading from 'the book' and seemed to be talking about Fiona, who had already passed on. A little later in the month Mum also said, 'The new book I have is useful.' Now she is talking about eight books. This does indeed sound like the

Akashic Records of the Other World, in which all information throughout time is said to exist.

As I have already mentioned, and am witnessing with greater clarity as time goes by, the information Mum has given me over the last couple of years suggests that there are a number of different phases or stages of dying. Many spiritual and shamanic teachings talk about the passage from this life into the next, but Mum is describing these things while she is still here in this world. It would seem that she is able to access the Other World through her inner senses, her inner tele-vision, and choose what she wants to learn. If this is so, then she is giving me extraordinary insights into the Other World. What a truly amazing gift!

I refer to her out-of-body travel and her recent visit to her brother, and she says again, 'I don't want to do too much.' When I talk to her about her astral body and its relation to her aura, Mum responds without any prompting and says, 'mental'. In esoteric philosophy the mental body is above the astral body, having a higher frequency than the physical body and the emotional astral body.

Evening. Mum is in bed and bright eyed. She is observing me, as she does.

Mum: *Your skin needs more white, Margaret.*
Me: *You are absolutely right. Well observed, Mum.*

I elaborate a little on this subject, drawing on my knowledge of Traditional Chinese Medicine (TCM) to explain that my skin lacks white because of an imbalance in my body. I have never discussed this with Mum but her observation is absolutely correct and supports this diagnostic aspect of TCM.

Mum: *Margaret knows a lot. Fiona and Emily never had times like this.*

I know about things that interest me. These particular subjects have never been of interest to Fiona or Emily.

Mum: *There are many centuries. I don't know which one – difficult.*
I want to write to people.
Me: *Who do you want to write to, Mum?*
No reply.

I am curious. This sounds to me like a reference to past lives. Could her observation have arisen out of her accessing the library, the eight books and the history contained in them? Psychics say information about past lives is held in the Akashic Records. They also say, as do people who have had a near-death experience (NDE), that in other dimensions linear time does not exist – something that is hard for us in the physical world to comprehend.

Mum: ... *flask* [touching her throat]. *I need to get the balance right.*
I have worked hard. It's been fun. This is a lovely holiday.

I'm so glad Mum is experiencing my visits as a holiday. Strange though it may sound, they feel like that for me, too. Because I am not with her all the time, when I am it is intense and very special. This is one reason why I continue with this pattern of visiting.

Saturday 28 May 2005

Mum is in her room. It is 11am and Paul is with me.

Mum: *This isn't fair to Paul.*
Paul: *I like seeing you, Granny. I do, really.*

I think she feels that Paul, being in his twenties, shouldn't have to spend his time in this way. However he is mature and cares deeply about her, so is very happy to be visiting her. Aware of the special relationship Mum and I enjoy, and not quite knowing where he fits in, he doesn't say very much. For this reason I encourage him to visit her without me being present.

Mum: *I want William's address.*

I think she wants to know how she can reach Dad, which may mean connecting with him at a different level, so I need to arrange for them to meet on their own and have some quality time together. Although Dad frequently visits Mum in the care home, his visits are brief and take place in the public arena of the residents' lounge. Maybe Mum requires a special private meeting.

Evening. Mum is in bed and in a reflective mood.

Mum: *We* [she and I] *had a difficult beginning but we've had a good ending.*
Me: *Yes, it's amazing how we've worked through everything. I'm so grateful.*
Mum: *Margaret has a lot of knowledge. Margaret is good.*
Me: *Thank you, Mum, so have you.*
    I see you keep moving your head from left to right and back again.
Mum: *I'm keeping both brains active.*
Me: *That's a good exercise for that. You're doing really well.*

Speaking as a kinesiologist, such movements are indeed one way of activating both hemispheres of the brain. She seems to know intuitively what to do or maybe she is receiving instructions from the Other World.

Mum: *Emily and William don't have this* [i.e. this understanding and shared knowledge].

139

Mum makes a further reference to 'the night has many nights' and 'the whole world' but gives no explanation when I ask her.

Me: *Do you remember me when I am not here?*
Mum: *Yes, Margaret.*

Wednesday 22 June 2005

It is Mum's ninetieth birthday today and I am back to celebrate with her. Another year and she is still here. As always, I give her a bunch of sweet peas.

Me: *Hello Mum. Happy Birthday! How are you on this special day?*
Mum: *Fine, thank you.*

She has a lovely day with cards and presents. The cook at the care home has made a cake for her and all the staff make her feel very special.

The weather is fine so in the afternoon Mum, Dad, Emily, a few family friends and I have tea on the lawn at our house.

Evening. Mum is in bed and quiet. She is looking at me in prolonged silence.

Mum: *What's stopping you?*

This is such a pertinent question, one I am also asking myself. Having just arrived, and after all the activities of the day, I am not yet fully connected with her and am having difficulty staying in sustained, silent eye contact. To make it harder for me, these eye-gazing sessions are getting longer owing to Mum's brain activity slowing down. I need to shift from my chattering 'monkey mind' into a state of mindfulness. I find it helps if I listen to the silence and become an observer of myself.

Thursday 23 June 2005

It is a lovely morning so I take Mum out in the wheelchair along the promenade. The care home is always very hot and stuffy so the fresh sea air is good for us.

Evening. Mum is in her room.

Me: *What are you thinking?*

I can see from her facial expression that she is processing information.

Mum: *I can't remember. I'm enjoying your company.*
Me: *Yes, Mum, it's just lovely being together like this.*

Saturday 26 June 2005

It is a fine day again so we have another morning outing in the wheelchair. The schools are on holiday now, so there are lots of children and young families around. People are very friendly and Mum engages with everyone we encounter as we progress very slowly along the promenade. Later, in the residents' lounge:

Me: *You're looking very bright, Mum.*
Mum: *You're here, Margaret.*
Me: *Oh, Mum, you are lovely.*

These straightforward, joyful words gladden my heart.

Evening. We are together in her room.

Mum: *I want to be fair to William.*

It seems she is still having some difficulty with Dad, but I don't know exactly what she is concerned about. In an attempt to help, I offer to talk with her about their lives together and she is eager to do this. Afterwards she says she feels better, so it seems she has gained some insights and new ways of seeing and thinking about their relationship. I am amazed at how open and responsive she is.

Mum: *I'm in my little turret and very happy.*

This comment suggests she feels safe and contained; interesting, as it follows on from our talking about her and Dad. Incidentally, my surname, La Tourelle, means 'turret' (literally, 'little tower') in French.

Sunday 27 June 2005

Fortunately, we are having a good spell of weather, so we have another morning outing in the wheelchair. Mum is concerned that pushing her might be too much for me but I assure her it isn't. I enjoy these outings. Despite all the logistical difficulties, they are such a lovely way to spend time together. Her interest in everything we encounter slows me down and we have time to amble along and just be. It is like a mindfulness meditation. What a luxury in this modern world.

Evening. Mum is in her room.

Mum: *I'm thinking of all the things I'd like to do.*
Me: *What would you like to do, Mum? Tell me.*
Mum: *I'd like to fly.*
Me: *Good! We can do that. Shall we have a little practice? Know that you can come back whenever you wish, right here with me.*

I offer her this visualization:

> *Now, when you are ready, close your eyes.*
> *Let everything slow down, very slow.*

*Imagine you are as light as a feather and you start to lift off
    and up effortlessly.*
Feel yourself floating in space.
Enjoy feeling totally weightless and free.
Floating in this timeless space.
*Gently moving in space or just hovering. And take as long as
    you want ...*
*Now, very gently, in your own time, float back down again,
    gently, gently.*
Feel the weight of your body starting to rest in the chair.
When you are ready, open your eyes.
Be aware of being in the room here with me.
Take your time.

Me: *Did you enjoy that?*
Mum: *Yes, that was wonderful, Margaret.*

My short guided visualization enabled Mum, if only briefly, to
enjoy the sense of freedom that she was seeking.

Sunday 31 July 2005

It is a few weeks since I have seen Mum and I am back for Dad's
birthday tomorrow. Mum is in her room, looking bright. She
is wearing a newly acquired white jumper from the care home
collective wardrobe, not the most flattering colour against her
very pale complexion.

Me: *Hello Mum. It's lovely to see you again. How are you?*
      How are you feeling?
Mum: *Fine, thank you, Margaret.*

For some time she talks, often repeating what she has just said.
Then she says:

Mum: [Emphatically] *Choice. It's good to have choice.*
Me: *Yes it is. I agree. What would you like to have choice about?*
No reply.

Choice – this is one of the really big questions. Do we have choice and free will or don't we? Mum's statement, 'It's good to have choice' suggests that we can have choice but it is not automatic. I recall what she said last May about not wanting the new television programme – so she wasn't able to exercise choice then. But in February this year she said, 'I'm getting ready for the next programme. I need to decide which programme', indicating that she did have choice then. What enabled her to move from a position of not having choice to one in which she has choice? Might it have been as a result of the learning she gained from the programmes and the tests and supervision she underwent? If this is so, it seems we should not fear the tests that life presents to us but should embrace them and view them as an opportunity to learn and to move toward gaining greater choice and free will.

I wonder what she wants to have choice about now? Can she see something that is prompting this statement?

Mum: *I want everything to be in order. I like things to be tidy.*

She has talked before about her need for order and there is nothing unusual about someone at the end of life wanting this. However, her need might be arising from an attempt to deal with the increasing disorder that she is experiencing as her brain function declines.

Monday 1 August 2005

Morning.

Mum: [Emphatically, as I kiss her goodbye] *You'll love it. You'll love it.*

Is she talking about the Other World? I choose to believe she is and feel greatly reassured. In fact I feel more than reassured; it is absolutely wonderful to know this. The information Mum has been passing on to me is very liberating and is giving me a new perspective on dying that is also changing how I experience living.

Afternoon. It is Dad's birthday. Mum's mood is a little flat but lightens at this:

Dad: *I really admire the way you are coping with this, Pat. It can't be easy.*
Mum: *Thank you for your support, William. I couldn't have done it without you.*

It is the first time I have heard either of them truly acknowledge the other and my heart is filled with relief and joy. What a beautiful birthday present.

I think Dad is learning, maybe as a result of his 'operation' and what Mum has passed on to him on an energetic level. Everything seems to be moving along nicely.

Evening.

Mum: *Your eyes are so brown. Your eyes sparkle. I'm taking the eyes but you will remember them. Lots of memories, so many!*
Me: *What do you mean? Tell me about the eyes, Mum. Tell me about your memories.*
No reply.

I wonder what the memories are. And 'the eyes', what a mysterious thing to say! I am totally bewildered and bewitched.

Mum: *The surgery has been very well done.*
Me: *I'm pleased to hear that. You certainly seem well.*

She has made several references to operations in the past. Whatever mysterious forces are at work, they appear to be helping her on all levels, physical, emotional, mental and spiritual. She is much better than I would have expected her to be at this severe stage of Alzheimer's disease.

Mum: *I want to get up.*
Me: *Good, let's do it. Let's imagine getting up.*

Of course she can't actually get up. I do some visualization with her again. Helping her to fulfil imaginatively the desires that she can't fulfil physically gives her a brief escape from her bodily limitations. It also helps to reinforce the belief that what you think or imagine is what you get.

Mum: *That was lovely, Margaret.*
        Your hair is loose. Your hair shines. You are so brown.
        I'm doing well. I'm a battler.
Me: *Yes you are. Well done, Mum. You deserve a medal.*

Tuesday 2 August 2005

Morning. It is another lovely day so we go for a wheelchair walk along the promenade. The sun is shining and there is a soft southwesterly breeze blowing off the sea. We can hear the joyful sounds of children playing on the beach, their shrieks of delight as they splash at the water's edge. There is a queue at the kiosk where we stop to buy ice cream. I hadn't anticipated the challenges eating this might present on a hot day. A kind passer-by, seeing my predicament, comes to my rescue with a handful of tissues. Things are constantly changing with Alzheimer's and every new situation presents a new challenge. It is hard keeping up.

Evening. Mum is in bed. She says she is tired.

Mum: *It's lovely having you here, Margaret.*
Me: *You know I love being here with you.*
What are you thinking about, Mum?
Mum: *The future. What is going to happen? I'm thinking a lot.*
My thinking has improved.

I believe this – I can see she is thinking a lot. Her eyes are closed, her head is turning from side to side and her expression is changing. The problem is that her ability to remember what she has just thought, and to put it into words, is decreasing.

Regarding the future and what is going to happen, she knows more about this than me and I'm sure she will tell me when the time is right.

Mum: *I'm helping Emily to become a person in her own right.*
Me: *Good. That is lovely. Just right!*

It would seem that help for Emily is coming, through Mum, possibly from Emily's mum, Fiona, in the Other World. And I am Mum's companion and witness. This shows the energy dynamics and healing ripple effect of our family constellation at work in a most amazing way.

Mum: *William, he tried hard.*

This is true and I am so glad that she is acknowledging this now. She then moves on to Margaret and me.

Mum: *Margaret and you* [me] *are very different.*
Me: *Margaret, is that me?*
Mum: *Yes.*
Me: *Are Margaret and me the same?*
Mum: *Yes.*
Me: *Can you explain the two of us?*
Mum: *I can't explain the differences.*

The mystery of Margaret and me continues.

147

Wednesday 3 August 2005

Morning. The matron and I are talking about Mum and how surprised we both are at how well she can still communicate, considering the advanced stage of her Alzheimer's. For over a year now Mum has been taking a daily herbal complex, which has been prescribed for her by a medical doctor and herbalist. The matron believes this is what has made the difference.

Mum is up, sitting in a chair and looking fine. She has had her hair done by the visiting hairdresser. We chat about this and that.

Evening. Mum is in bed. As she can't move to reposition herself, she now has a special pressure-relief mattress. This contains lots of internal chambers in which the air pressure is constantly changing, to avoid bed sores. As I lie on the bed alongside her I feel a very strange sensation of movement in different places under my body. I wonder what it feels like for her. She hasn't commented on it.

Mum: *You have strong legs. You have clever hands.*
      Margaret and you are so different.
Me: *In what way are we different?*
Mum: *I can't say how.*
      [After some thought] *I didn't want to spoil, upset ...*
      your birthday.

What a strange thing to say. She didn't spoil or upset my birthday. I am puzzled by this remark.

Mum: *Margaret has fixed the gas.*

This is true and another example of her clairvoyance – the fourth! How does she know this? I haven't told her that last night I mended the gas fire in the front room of our house. She didn't say, 'You fixed the gas'; she said, 'Margaret fixed the gas.' This suggests, as I suspected, that she is meeting me and tapping into

148

Mum: *Margaret phones me. She keeps in touch. I may not stay for long. Margaret's number is 31260 and lots of numbers.*

This is yet another reminder that she will not be here for ever. It is true I phone her nearly every day when I am away.

The number she quoted is very close to our house telephone number. She was always good at remembering telephone numbers.

Wednesday 14 September 2005

Evening. I am back after a break. Mum is in bed, drifting in and out of sleep.

Mum: *You have a loving face. I see it in your face. You have lovely hair, nice shoulders, lovely teeth.*
Me: *Thank you, Mum.*
Mum: *All right, life is difficult. We all get old. We have to move on.*
I don't want to leave you.
Me: *You'll never leave me. We may not always be together in this world but in spirit we will be together, always, in an Other World.*

I feel tears welling up in me as I say this.

Mum: *You let me probe your mind. I thank you for that.*

When we talk about this I feel such closeness. It is absolutely true and it hasn't been easy for me. Probing is exactly what it feels like when she stares at me with her unfaltering gaze, without words. My mind is still racing having just arrived from London and I am feeling uncomfortable, as if I am trying to escape from myself.

Because Mum has Alzheimer's, she is totally open to me and can engage in this prolonged stillness with attention. I try to be open to her, transparent even, and let her 'probe my mind', as she calls it. I wonder if our willingness to be accessible to each other is allowing information from the Other World, that would otherwise be blocked, to enter our shared sacred space.

Mum: *There is a man comes to me – the mysteries of life.*
Me: *Who is he? Tell me about him.*
Mum: *I don't know.*

I want to know more but she has moved on. This sounds like another visitor from the Other World. I wonder about the purpose of his visits.

I talk to her about our journey over the last two years: the revelations and how healing it has been for both of us.

Me: *How are things between you and Dad?*
Mum: *Very good, very good.*

This is the first time I have ever heard her say this, and it is an amazing new position to have reached, especially at this stage in their lives. About four months ago she said she was helping him and that seems to be benefiting them both. I feel a great sense of relief. I have been praying for them to find resolution before they die.

Mum: *My mother and father, they are there. The little skinny one.* [She was the little skinny one.] *I've lost my looks.*

So she is continuing to keep in touch with her relatives in the Other World.

Me: *You are still beautiful. Your eyes are so blue. They search for the truth. You still look the same to me.*
Mum: *Goodbye, it's the time.*

154

Oh! My heart misses a beat. Is this really it or yet another rehearsal?

Stopping for a moment and putting myself in her position, I realize that while she is drifting between the two worlds, she may well experience leaving this one as she slips into the other one.

DEEPENING CONNECTION

'The lost roses.'
Pat

Thursday 15 September 2005

Evening. Mum is in bed.

Mum: *I'm in my new home. Call me the cleanser.*

Yesterday she said 'goodbye' and today she has moved to her 'new home'. So it sounds as if she has made the move, possibly the one she said she was preparing for back in December 2003. Reflecting on her many announcements about leaving and about choice, I wonder now if she has had a choice about whether to leave or stay, and has decided to stay. Or was she talking about leaving one phase or stage of the dying process and moving on to a new one, rather than finally departing from this life? If I had thought about these possibilities before, I might have saved myself a lot of anguish. I am learning all the time.

Regarding cleansing, her probing my mind is deeply cleansing. I couldn't find a better word to describe it myself. Is she preparing me for deeper spiritual practice?

Me: *Yes, you are the cleanser. You have cleansed me and I thank you for it.*

Over time I have learned to surrender to Mum's silent gaze and am now able to stay with her probing my mind, without feeling any need to escape. Hallelujah!

Mum: *I may just slip away. No tears.*

> *Emily is lively. See that she is sensible. Be fair.*

Me: *You know I will look after Emily and of course I will be fair.*

Mum: *I want to try to remember what it is to be normal. It has been wonderful having these moments together.*
You have an open face.

Me: *This is the result of you probing and cleansing me, Mum.*

Her course of probing and cleansing has been really tough, but it has been worth it. I feel much clearer now – it has helped me to move on.

I talk to her about her life, as it was when she was living at home, the daily routines, the cat and other things, focusing on the positive of course.

Friday 16 September 2005

Evening. Mum is sitting in her chair, looking bright. I am playing a CD of Mozart's piano concertos and giving her a manicure. It is a truly lovely evening. There are no searching questions – just a practical reminder of what is *normal*.

Mum: *We are much closer now, Margaret, unlike before.*

Me: *Yes we are and it's just lovely, Mum. It makes me feel very happy, too.*

More silent tears!

In these moments she still remembers the feelings and can compare past and present.

Saturday 17 September 2005

Evening. Mum is awake and looking thoughtful.

Mum: *I'm thinking of William. How is he?*

Me: *He's fine. He struggles on.*

Mum: *I want to send a message to Margaret. Margaret needs to take time for herself.*

Margaret needs to listen. What Mum is saying is absolutely true. Dad is in need of more and more support and I am trying to manage this to his high standards, often from a distance. I think she is sensing the stress this is causing in me. This is another example of her tuning in to me.

Mum: *I'm alive!*

Her eyes were closed and as she opens them she sounds surprised that she is still here. Maybe she drifted off into the Other World and has come back again.

Me: *I need to go back to London to work, but as you know I will be back with you again soon.*
Mum: *Do you want to work?*
Me: *Yes, I enjoy what I do.*
Mum: [With affection] *You haven't changed.*

As well as seeing clients for therapy, I run training courses in London that extend over a period of six months. Students make their arrangements, such as booking flights and hotels, months or even years ahead. I am feeling increasingly anxious about being able to meet my commitments to them. So far, thankfully, I have been able to.

Wednesday 12 October 2005

It is late afternoon and I have just arrived off the train from London.

Mum is in the lounge.

Me: *Hello Mum. It's lovely to see you again. How are you?*

Mum: *Fine.*

Evening. Mum is in bed in her room.

Mum: *Margaret has managed this well. She's come out of it well.*
Me: Yes I have. Thank you, Mum! You've helped me and I've
     gained so much.
Mum: *I'm better. I've made a wonderful recovery. It's the skill of
     the two women. They talk to me. I feel comfort. I'm alive.*

What a positive statement from someone who was diagnosed
with Alzheimer's disease five years ago.

At the beginning of our journey back in 2003, Mum told me
that two women were visiting her and helping her. These visitors
were not from this world and it sounds as if their help has been
on-going. How wonderful!

Later, very much in this world:

Mum: *I don't belong anywhere. I don't want to be out flat.*
     [She is lying flat in bed and can barely move.] *It doesn't
     suit me.*

This suggests she is experiencing two different states of
awareness: one an out-of-body existence that is wonderful; and
another in her physical body that is not 'normal' as she wants
it. At least she has some temporary relief from the physical
limitations from time to time.

Mum: *You have lovely teeth. Margaret is a wonderful dancer.
     You have a well-proportioned face.*

Mum often fixates on my face and particularly my teeth,
presumably because I am talking. I am playing music and
dancing around the room, as I do for her. I am not so sure about
'wonderful dancer', but maybe she is experiencing me dancing as
if she is dancing herself. I hope so.

Thursday 13 October 2005

Evening.

Mum: *I've everything organized. It's nearly complete. I think a lot.*

I have been practising maintaining my gaze into Mum's eyes as she stares at me and am no longer resisting this. What I am seeing now is just an absent look, but she is still here. I am expecting more but maybe this is it. Maybe she no longer has any need of a personal identity. Where is she?

In December 2003 she said, 'I am getting everything ready in a position for starting.' Now, nearly two years later, she is saying, 'It's nearly complete.' This suggests knowledge of the process of dying and of where she is in the process. She seems to know this at all levels: subconscious, conscious and superconscious.

Mum: *Tele-vision is amazing. I can ask all my questions.*

She is looking into the distance. What is she seeing? What is she asking in her mind? She has talked about her inner tele-vision, her portal to the Other World, on a number of occasions and has spoken about accessing programmes. (She doesn't watch TV.) Now she is describing the process as interactive. She can access any information she wants from the Other World. How amazing! Having this gift is meaningless unless you know what to ask for – and she does.

The CD player stops and suddenly, without any intervention, starts playing again. It is not unusual for electrical interference to occur in the presence of psychic energy and, given all that is happening, I wouldn't be surprised if this is the cause.

Mum: *My memory has gone. I don't have any brain cells left.*
Me: *That's not the case, Mum. If you had no brain cells, you wouldn't be able to say that. We're all losing brain cells*

*and this happens increasingly as we get older. You are
still you and I love you as you are.*
Mum: *I don't want to leave.*

Oh dear, I don't want her to leave, either. This journey together
has brought us so close. I am spending most of the time now
quietly holding her.

Mum: *I love you, Margaret. You were my first-born.*
Me: *I love you, too, Mum.*

I feel myself filling up with emotion – more silent tears.
      She speaks about Dad and his falls and struggle.

Mum: *It will all come right in the end.*

Friday 14 October 2005

Afternoon. I take Mum out in the car to our favourite beauty
spots. Again, by the evening she has forgotten. As I observed
before, this is all about being in the 'now', living in the moment.

Evening. We sing together, songs we know and love, such as 'My
Love is Like a Red, Red Rose' by Robert Burns.

Mum: *Don't leave it too long.*

Is this a message for me? I presume she means till I come back.

Saturday 15 October 2005

Evening.

Mum: *I need more fluids.*

Mum must have been very dehydrated, as she drank five glasses
of water one after the other. Every time I am with her I offer

her water and help her to drink it, which is a very slow process these days.

Me: *What are you thinking about?*
Mum: *Nothing.* [She hiccups] *When I hiccup I realize I'm still alive.*

This suggests she is losing her bodily sensory awareness and that more physical contact would be reassuring.

Wednesday 9 November 2005

It is only three weeks since I last saw Mum, but this time there is little voluntary communication from her. What has happened? Usually when I arrive she is very eager to talk, as if she has been storing up things to tell me.

Me: *Hello Mum. How are you?*
Mum: *Average.*
Me: *What are you thinking?*
Mum: *Nothing.*
        Your face is covered.

I don't wear foundation make-up. Am I hiding something? If I am I am not aware of it. She is wearing her reading glasses and I look at them. They are very smudged so no wonder what she is seeing is 'covered'. I don't know how long she has been seeing the world in this way. The care assistants don't always notice when her glasses are dirty and I can't count the number of times I have had to clean them.

Thursday 10 November 2005

Evening. Mum is in bed, looking bright.

Mum: *I don't like having nothing to do. It doesn't suit me.*

The fact that she knows she has nothing to do shows that she is aware.

Mum: *I've had an operation.*

She told me two years ago about operations that she said helped her and it seems these energetic healing interventions are continuing.

Me: *Have you? You've had a bladder infection but thankfully you're over that now.*

Mum: *You're a lovely girl. You have the right values. Don't do too much.*

She sent a message to Margaret before about taking time for herself. Margaret and I need to pay more attention to this.

We hum along to *Clair de Lune*. She is happy.

Me: *Dream of dancing, lovely Mummy.*

Friday 11 November 2005

Mum is in bed. We return to *The Prophet* and I select the poem on teaching. Mum reads this enthusiastically and comments on it. She is so delighted to be able to do this. These poems are perfect for her as they are short but also have deep meaning.

I searched through our books at home to find some that would stimulate her long-term memory and I came across a childhood favourite: *Fairies of the Flowers and Trees* by Cicely Mary Barker. This is a beautifully illustrated book with very sweet poems. We take our time looking at the pictures and reminiscing. When Fiona was little we called her the Scilla Fairy because she had the same fair hair and blue eyes. Mum and I read this poem together and remember Fiona as that dear, innocent little girl.

Mum: *Little Fiona.*

Little Fiona passed on six years ago. What a sad life. But she is in a better place now and, thankfully, helping us all.

We hum together to *Clair de Lune* again. Lovely.

Saturday 12 November 2005

Evening. Mum is sitting in a chair and I am giving her a manicure. The care assistants are so busy this is something that can get overlooked, but it is a very nice pastime for us. It is good to do normal things like this together.

Then we read more poems from *Fairies of the Flowers and Trees* and look at the illustrations. A care assistant brings in tea and we enjoy this together and have a loving hug.

Mum: *I love your company.*
Me: *Yes, it's lovely being together.*
I want to tell you what Dad said to me. He said that he realizes now that you've had a difficult life with many family deaths and he didn't show you the understanding he should have done at the time. He regrets this.

Mum hears this and I can see she looks comforted. It is part of the journey my parents are on as they approach the end of their lives and strive to heal their past.

Christmas Day 2005

We are all here for Christmas, Paul, Emily and I, and are engaged in lots of festive activities.

As usual, I encourage Paul and Emily to visit their granny without me. It is so busy over this holiday period that there is no quiet time for Mum and me to be together in our special way.

2006

New Year's Day 2006

Evening. Mum is in bed, alternating between alertness and drifting off.

Mum: *You have nice hands. You feel warm. What makes your hands feel so warm?*
Me: *It's energy. This happens when I'm feeling the energy flowing.*
Mum: *That's lovely.*

She is feeling the energy connection between us.

Mum: *I see the energy coming out of your face. I don't often see that.*

She is seeing my aura and most likely the energy coming from my brow chakra (the energy centre positioned between the eyebrows). This is yet another new skill she has acquired. She lifts her hand and touches my brow on the left.

Me: *What are you doing?*
Mum: *I'm tidying it up.*
Me: *Thank you.*

This is an unusual gesture; other than moving her head from side to side, she doesn't move much now. Maybe my energy needed a little tidying up.

Mum: *You have colour in your face. Do you have rouge on your cheeks?*
Me: *No.*
Mum: *You look healthy.*
Me: *That's good. I sometimes worry about my health.*

Mum: *You have no need to.*
      I see lots of pictures.
Me: *What kind of pictures?*
No reply.
Mum: *You're lovely.*
Me: *Thank you, Mum. So are you.*
      I'm going away tomorrow, Mum. I'm really sorry to be leaving you.

Every time I am in this situation, about to leave Mum, I question what I am doing. However, spending time back in London means that while I am here I can give Mum my undivided attention, something I could not do if I was here constantly. I need to have a break so that I can come back refreshed and engage with the intense focus that enables us to enter deeply into our sacred space.

Mum: *Oh that's a pity. When will you be back?*
Me: *In a few weeks.*

Tears are again welling up in my eyes.

Monday 2 January 2006

Me: *I'm leaving for the train now Mum, but you know I will be back soon.*

As I travel back to London on the train, whenever I think about Mum feelings well up inside me and tears start to roll down my cheeks. This is really hard for me.

———————————————

I am back in Scotland again and thinking how very fortunate I am to experience the contrast between the busy metropolis and this very pleasant place by the sea. Walking along the beach for miles with no one around is like a meditation. It is where I go to ask the *big* questions and allow the answers to come. Gazing out at distant horizons and breathing in the pure sea air feeds my soul. I feel completely at home in myself.

Wednesday 1 February 2006

I have been back a few days and have been visiting Mum. It is evening and she is in her room.

Me: *Hello Mum. It's lovely to see you again. How are you feeling?*
Mum: *Fair.*

As I kiss her I notice that her neck feels very warm, and I comment on this.

Mum: *It's stuck, full up.*

I think her glands are swollen and she has a fever. I alert the staff nurse.

Thursday 2 February 2006

Mum seems to be a bit better today and is in her room, looking thoughtful.

Mum: *I have lots of thoughts.*
Me: *What thoughts? Tell me.*
Mum: *I can't, my brain doesn't work.*
Me: *Does that bother you?*
Mum: *No, not at all. I don't have any worries.*
Me: *That's good.*

She is telling me her thoughts are not coming from her brain, but they need to be processed by her brain in order for her to be able to speak and tell me about them.

Friday 3 February 2006

Evening. Mum is in bed and we are singing songs by Robert Burns together.

Mum: *He must have loved very deeply.*

We are sitting silently, looking at each other. She appears to be trying to say something.

Me: *You have something to say to me?*
Mum: *I don't know what it is.*
Me: *What do you see?*

I wonder if a visual prompt might help.

Mum: *William. I don't remember anything.*

She had Dad in mind after commenting, 'He must have loved deeply.' I wonder if she was thinking about their marriage.

Me: *Mum, do you remember me when I was a little girl?*

I ask this question as she said, 'I don't remember anything', but I know she can access her long-term memory more easily.

Mum: *Yes, Margaret.*
Me: *So you can remember.*
Mum: *Yes.*
Me: *You are fine.*
Mum: *Am I?*

She looks pleased. As she had a memory blank, I wanted to activate her memory to reassure her and boost her confidence – and it seems that this worked.

Saturday 4 February 2006

Morning. Mum is in her room and I am sitting quietly by her side holding her hand.

Me: *What are you thinking, Mum?*
Mum: *I'm not thinking.*
Me: *How are you feeling?*
Mum: *I'm feeling a bit lost, Margaret.*

We look at old family photos and reminisce. This helps her to feel connected with her life again and not so lost.

Saturday 25 February 2006

Morning. It is a few weeks since I have seen Mum.

Me: *Hello Mum. It's lovely to see you again. How are you? How are you feeling?*
Mum: *Average.*

Mum is looking bright but is not able to communicate much in words. We are in the lounge with other people. The activities co-ordinator is leading a movement-to-music session and residents are joining in with various degrees of competency. Afterwards, I chat with some of the residents about everyday things.

Over the years, through my frequent visiting, I have become part of the care home community and it has become an important part of my life, too. I know the residents by name and engage with them each time I see them. I have also got to know members of staff and we chat about life, family things and health. Other regular visitors who, like me, have resident relatives, stop and chat. There is a general feeling of mutual respect and goodwill.

I have the utmost admiration for the staff and they are genuinely interested in what I do and my work in holistic healthcare. The proprietor even invited me to run workshops for the staff and this was so successful I did it a few times. I taught them how to look after themselves better, physically and emotionally, as they did their demanding work, and suggested how they could also apply this learning to residents. The unglamorous image of the residential care home often hides the reward of being part of the loving, caring community that works and lives within.

Me: *What are you thinking?*
Mum: *I don't know.*
Me: *What are you feeling?*
Mum: *I don't know.*
Me: *Are you happy?*
Mum: *Yes.*
Me: *Are you sad?*
Mum: *No.*
Me: *Good, it's fine.*
Mum: *It's amazing, Margaret. We're like twins.*

This is welcome confirmation that she feels included even though my attention has been with other residents. I asked her the questions about happiness and sadness to check that she isn't just saying 'yes' to everything. It seems this questioning has jogged her mind into action again.

Two years ago Mum said we had parallel thoughts and now she is saying we are like twins. This shows the closeness and similarity that she is sensing between us. Being like twins means our souls are connected at the spiritual level.

Monday 27 February 2006

Evening. Mum is in bed, I am giving her lots of stroking.

Mum: *That's lovely.*

170

We read more poems and look at illustrations from *Fairies of the Flowers and Trees*. Mum can read perfectly and this is very good for her morale.

Mum: *Margaret has discovered something wonderful.*

This is true. I know that she can read with meaning and pleasure, despite not being able to remember what she has just thought a moment ago.

Wednesday 29 March 2006

I have been here for a few days and have been visiting Mum regularly.

Me: *Hello Mum. How are you?*
Mum: *Fine.*

I notice that Mum's speech is a little less clear due to the muscles of her mouth not working so well and that she is dribbling down the right side. I wonder if she has had a little stroke and I mention this to the staff nurse.

Mum: *You're looking well, Margaret.*
Me: *Thank you. Are you happy, Mum?*
Mum: *Yes.*
Me: *Are you sad?*
Mum: *No.*
Me: *Do you have any pain?*
Mum: *No.*
Me: *Good, it's fine.*

She is initiating conversation less frequently now but can answer yes or no. As before, I use these basic questions to check that she is not in any discomfort. They are also a way to activate her brain and open the possibility of a conversation.

I am continuing to record our conversations in this late stage of Alzheimer's, not because they are full of revelations like before, but because they are an important record of the process of the disease.

Me: *What are you thinking?*
Mum: *How to find a way out.*
Me: *Do you want a way out now?*
Mum: *No.*
Me: *Would you like to go out?*

I know what she means but I want to create a way out, albeit one in this world.

Mum: *Yes.*
Me: *We could go out in the car this afternoon.*
Mum: *You're a lovely girl. Don't feel sad.*

I am feeling upset. It is hard for me to see her struggling, wanting a way out of this life and at the same time wanting to be here with me.

Afternoon. We go out in the car to our familiar places. The wind is blowing and the clouds are low and heavy with rain. The sea looks grey and choppy and sea gulls swoop and dive. The Isle of Arran is barely visible. Then we turn inward to the shelter of the woods where children play.

While we are sitting in the car, I tell Mum about my son Paul who is now in New York working as an architect on the 9/11 Memorial Museum Pavilion at the World Trade Center site.

Mum: *He needs to be careful.*

I have been feeling anxious about him being there and she has just confirmed my fear. There is nothing I can do to ease my

172

worry. My son, my only son, has to lead his own life and make his own choices. I trust that his intuition and inner knowing will guide him.

Evening. Mum is in bed and looking bright.

Mum: *It's a pleasure to see you, Margaret.*
Me: *It's a pleasure to see you, Mum.*

I am holding Mum's hand and thinking about the Mother's Day card I sent her. Where is it? It should be sitting on top of her chest of drawers but I can't see it. Oh dear, I don't think she received it. I feel sad. I made it for her, wanting her to know that I was remembering her on Mother's Day, even though I couldn't be with her. Unfortunately, these things happen in care homes. It was a paper collage of twelve red roses, all meticulously cut out and pasted on a card.

Mum: *The lost roses.*

Amazing! She has picked up not only the image but also the fact that the card has been lost. We are indeed like twins. This is a telepathic communication and the fifth example of her tuning in and her ESP. I tell her about the card I wanted her to have from me and we talk about our very special connection and her gift of telepathy.

As I leave she waves happily to me without any prompting. This has been a lovely hour together. I leave her with the CD of *Clair de Lune* playing on repeat.

Thursday 30 March 2006

Morning. I visit Mum briefly and give her a kiss.

Mum: *You've made my day, Margaret.*

Evening. Mum is in bed.

Mum: *I'm enjoying myself.*
Me: *Good. You look happy.*

Being with her now is not necessarily about long conversations but more about frequent contact. I am finding, unlike before, that I am now the storyteller. Given her wisdom, it seems appropriate at this time in her life to be talking about philosophical and spiritual matters. She enjoys listening to me and takes it all in.

I read to her from one of my favourite little booklets, *The Aloha Spirit* by Serge Kahili King. It summarizes the principles of Huna, the ancient Polynesian philosophy, which include: 'The world is what you think it is' and 'Energy flows where attention goes'. Mum understands instantly and enjoys this. These teachings have influenced my thinking and work over many years.

Lying beside her, I hug her as I tell her I am her daughter and that at the very beginning half of my genes came from her. We both marvel at this. Lots of Aloha Blessings.

Friday 31 March 2006

It is morning and Mum seems fine.

Mum: *You need to take it easy, moving house. You need to take it easy, Margaret.*

Psychic again! This is the sixth time she has tuned in to me at an extrasensory level. I have major building works going on in my London flat at the moment and am feeling very stretched trying to manage these while in Scotland.

Mum: *I'm taking up your time.*

Well observed, Mum. Although I am with her in person I am preoccupied thinking about my building project, so am not totally present. She senses this immediately.

Afternoon. We are in the residents' lounge drinking tea and eating homemade cakes. I ask her if she wants to go out but she says no.

Evening.

Mum: *You have a lovely face.*
I have lots of thoughts.

She isn't able to tell me what they are, however.

Wednesday 26 April 2006

It is a few weeks since I have seen Mum and she is in her room.

Me: *Hello Mum. It's lovely to see you again. How are you?*
Mum: *I'm fine.*
Me: *What are you thinking?*
Mum: *Lots of things.*
Me: *Tell me.*
Mum: *About life.*
Me: *What about life?*
Mum: *About leaving. I'm happy here.*
Me: *If you're happy here you will be happy anywhere, here and in the Other World.*
Is there anything you want from me?
Mum: *Your company.*
Me: *You will have it, dear Mummy. I am here now for a while.*

How direct and immediate. I am so pleased I am with her now.

It is interesting that there are times when Mum can put her thoughts into words, as she is doing today, and other times when she finds that difficult. This indicates intermittent disruption in parts of her brain.

Thursday 27 April 2006

Mum and I have lunch together in the care home. It is good to do this occasionally as it makes life seem more normal.

Mum: *It is nice to have your company, Margaret.*

Afternoon. We have an outing in the car.

Evening.

Mum: *You have a lovely face, Margaret.*
Me: *So have you, Mum*
Mum: *I can't remember what I am thinking.*
Forty-eight hours, that will do me. I can't remember.
Me: *It's not important. There only is now. Remembering is past.*

We sing together and I dance to the music.

Friday 28 April 2006

Morning. Mum is in her room and I am giving her a manicure and hand massage.

Evening.

Mum: *It's all done. Your cheeks have filled out.*

Has she told me everything? Right at the beginning of our journey, back in 2003, she said she would 'fill both cheeks'. She has remembered this and has fulfilled her promise – my cheeks have been 'filled out'. Now I do have lots of nourishing things to say. And that is an understatement!

I tell her about what is happening with Dad, Emily and Paul.

Mum: *How is Fiona?*
Me: *I know you know, Mum, that Fiona passed on some years ago. But she is with us in the Other World.*
Mum: *Oh yes, I know.*

She hasn't forgotten Fiona. That is nice.

I am giving her lots of quiet hugs with no thinking and no speaking.

Mum: *That was lovely. That was just lovely. You lifted the books.*

A year ago she made a reference to eight books. Maybe just being hugged lovingly, with no thinking or doing, has given her a break from her study, lifted a weight from her. I note that this way of being with her may be more appropriate now than entering into deep conversations as we have done in the past.

Saturday 29 April 2006

Afternoon. I bring Mum round to our home for tea. She struggles to cope gracefully. Later in the day she says:

Mum: *I am sorry you are going.*
Me: *Is there anything you need?*
Mum: *Me.*

I put my arm round her and we talk about the good times we have had together.

Is she saying she needs to find herself, or could it be me she needs? Whichever it is, her pleading eyes are heart-breaking. I ask myself if I am doing the right thing, coming and going. Should I be here all the time? If so I would need to have a life of my own. I could cope with the situation with Mum but I could not also deal with Dad being totally dependent on me. Their level of need is like a bottomless pit. Once here I would not be able to leave and that could go on for years. As it is, when I go out on an errand, I return to find Dad sitting at the window anxiously looking out for me, having imagined something terrible has happened.

I could not witness their distress and not respond to it. If I were part of a large extended family that could share the care, I would be very happy to stay. But on my own, I would find it overwhelming over time and it would be hard to remain positive. This is the price we pay in our modern world for having small families and so much mobility. What am I to do?

Friday 5 May 2006

Morning.

Me: *How are you?*
Mum: *I'm fine.*
Me: *What are you thinking?*
Mum: *Nothing.*
Me: *Is that all right?*
Mum: *Yes.*
Me: *What are you feeling?*
Mum: *Nothing.*
Me: *No pain?*
Mum: *No.*
Me: *Fine.*

Evening. Mum is in bed. I lie down and hug her. We don't speak much but she keeps looking at me.

Saturday 6 May 2006

Morning. I pop in for a brief visit. Now it is all about connecting, even if just to say hello.

Afternoon. We have a wheelchair walk to the sea front, then to the garden of our house for tea. It is a lovely outing.

Evening.

Mum: *Margaret is more patient.*

I hadn't been feeling impatient but maybe over the years Margaret has become more patient.

Sunday 7 May 2006

Morning. I pay Mum a quick visit.

Evening. Mum is still up in the lounge. She looks bright and relaxed and sounds very happy and contented. When I arrive she says without prompting:

Mum: *Hello Margaret!*

I am holding her hand.

Mum: *It's so lovely, holding your hand.*

Sunday 21 May 2006

Morning. I have just arrived after being in London for a couple of weeks.

Me: *Hello Mum. It's lovely to see you. How are you?*
Mum: *Average.*

Afternoon.

Mum: *I'm thinking about leaving.*

She has said this so many times before and I know what she means, but I want to check out all the possibilities.

Me: *Where would you like to go, home* [next door], *out?*
Mum: *No, I don't think so. There is no hurry.*
Me: *Everything in its own time.*

I realize there is no need for me to ask these facile questions any
more. We both know what she is talking about. She will leave in
her own time.

We are chatting about things when she says:

Mum: *My Mini* [her car].

In London the previous day a friend asked where I was going,
so I zoomed in on an aerial photo of my parents' house on my
computer to show him. There, to my surprise, sitting in the
driveway was Mum's old Mini. Her car had been sold years ago
when she was no longer fit to drive so the photo was clearly out
of date. I am keeping count of these psychic episodes – this is
the seventh.

Evening.

Mum: *Margaret works it all out.*
Me: *Is that good?*
Mum: *Yes.*
    Margaret has gone.

I had indeed gone; I was thinking of something else. I realize
that our space is sacred because of the loving feelings we have
toward each other and the way we are both totally present when
we're together in that space.

Mum: *You have lovely eyes. I see love in your eyes.*
Me: *Yes, I love you, Mum.*

Did she pick up on my thought about love, now that my attention
is back with her after I realized it had temporarily gone?

Monday 22 May 2006

Morning.

Mum: [Observing me, as she does] *You are well proportioned.*
Me: *Thank you, Mum.*

Evening.

Mum: *He doesn't know.*
Me: *Who doesn't know? What doesn't he know?*
No reply.

I imagine the 'he' she is talking about is Dad. But he is still in this world, so she would normally have answered a question relating to him. Is he here or is he, too, in the Other World now?

Mum: *We have the perfect arrangement, Margaret.*
Me: *Yes we do, Mum. It's wonderful.*
Mum: *I love your eyes.*
Me: *I love you, all of you.*

More loving hugs.

Wednesday 24 May 2006

Evening. Mum is resting in bed and I hug her without talking much. She nevertheless is looking at me intently.

Mum: *I'm very tired.*

I hold her hand and connect with the light. She is teaching me to be present. Her hand feels very light and fragile as if it has hardly any substance now. Silent tears.

Thursday 25 May 2006

Morning. I make a brief visit just to say hello and give her a kiss.

Afternoon. I take Dad in to see her and leave them alone in her room. I want to give them time together and the opportunity to deepen the connection that is growing between them at the end of their lives.

Evening.

Me: *Do you know you're still teaching me?*
        What do you think you're teaching me?

I want her to know that, although she isn't able to converse much, she is still of great value.

Mum: *Faith?*
Me: *Yes Mum, you have taught me faith.*
Mum: *You have such loving eyes.*
        We have had such precious moments.

I stop and take a deep breath and feel this deep in my heart and soul.

Me: *Yes we have and I'm so grateful.*
        You're totally present. Your memory is not good but you know everything in the moment. Dad says you're very calm and an example to us all.

Mum smiles softly. This affirmation from her husband is very important to her.

Friday 26 May 2006

It is the evening and Mum is still in the lounge when I arrive and is the last resident to go to bed. She says it's 'elastic'. I think she wanted to say 'flexible' but couldn't remember the word, so she used the closely associated word 'elastic' instead.

Me: *I know your memory is not very good but it seems to me you still think a lot. Is that so?*

Mum: *Yes.*

Saturday 27 May 2006

I take Mum out in the car to our special place where we look at the sea. This is very familiar and we enjoy just sitting and being silent as we take in the view and breathe in the fresh air.

Wednesday 21 June 2006

Morning. I am back again as it is Mum's birthday tomorrow.

Me: *Hello Mum. It's lovely to see you. How are you? How are you feeling?*

Mum: *Fine.*

      You're rushing.

She is right. I have just arrived from London and have been rushing and am still rushing. I need to be reminded of this. Actually, Margaret and I both need to pay more attention to this.

Evening. We are in the lounge. There is a lot of noise from the TV and people enjoying cups of tea and chattering. I am talking to people and Mum is enjoying being part of it all.

Mum: *That's nice.*

I am pleased she is able to be part of the social gathering and doesn't feel left out because she can't say much.

Thursday 22 June 2006

It is Mum's ninety-first birthday. Another year, another birthday, and Mum is still here.

Me: *What's it like being ninety-one?*
Mum: *I'd rather not think about it.*

What a thoughtless question of mine. I am clearly still not tuned in.

Me: *How are you feeling?*
Mum: *Fine.*
Me: *What are you thinking?*
Mum: *I don't know.*

Afternoon. I bring Mum to our house for a birthday tea on the lawn. Mum, Dad, Emily, a friend and I celebrate Mum's special day with her.

Evening. We are in the lounge.

Me: *What are you thinking, Mum?*
Mum: *The future.*
Me: *What about the future?*
No reply.

I am trying not to think about it but it is hard to imagine that she could go on for another year and have another birthday. She may be having the same thought.

Friday 7 July 2006

I am having little time with Mum as Dad is lurching from one crisis to another. He will be ninety-five in a few weeks and is trying, against all the odds, to be independent and remain in his own home. His mobility is poor and he is having frequent falls, but his mind is as sharp as ever. The current care arrangements are inadequate.

What am I going to do?

Tuesday 1 August 2006

It is Dad's ninety-fifth birthday. He is in good spirits and we have a birthday tea with the family, including my cousin (Dad's nephew) and a few friends. It is a relief to be in Scotland for a couple of weeks. During this time, I see Mum frequently but have nothing in particular to report.

Sunday 20 August 2006

I am still dealing with the escalating crisis with Dad, and as a result am not having much time with Mum. I explain the situation and she understands.

She is tuning in to me at the physical level:

Mum: *Margaret has weak tendons.*

I have weak ankles that could well be due to weak tendons.

Mum: [Emphatically] *Choice.*

Mum has used this word before but it seems to have a particular importance for her right now. I am wondering about the context in which she is saying this. What does she know? Choice about what I wonder?

Saturday 26 August 2006

There is a major new development today. Dad has a bad fall and breaks his elbow. Fortunately, I am here. He has emergency surgery and his arm is now in a plaster cast. His mobility was very poor before and now he can't do anything for himself and is going to require twenty-four-hour care.

I consider all the options and decide that the best one for him right now is to be in a home where there is nursing care. All the care homes in the area are full, including the one next door. In order for him to remain in the vicinity there is only one option – to move Mum from her single room into a shared room upstairs where, by chance, there is a spare bed. This would free up Mum's room for Dad. Because their relationship can be strained at times, putting them in the same room is not an option. I explain the situation to Mum and ask her if she would agree to move. The choice is hers, not mine. She agrees and the move takes place.

I know this arrangement is probably going to be permanent as there is no possibility of Dad living in his own home again. I feel desperately sad for him. This is another milestone. I am also very sad for Mum and me, as we have lost our private sacred space in which we have had such freedom for uninhibited expression and to explore the mysteries of this and the Other World. Her use a few days ago of the word 'choice' was indeed precognitive. I said that a bed was free 'by chance', but Jung believed, and I share this view, that there is no such thing as chance – this was synchronicity.

Thursday 31 August 2006

Mum: *You are wonderful, Margaret.*

This is a very stressful and difficult time for me, emotionally and practically. I know that Mum understands this. She couldn't have said anything nicer.

186

Mum: *You can remember things as they were.*

This is so true. How does she do it? Time and time again she finds exactly the right words to describe something. I sob quietly.

Friday 1 September 2006

I take Mum out in the car to have some one-to-one time together as we have not been able to do this since she moved into the shared room.

Me: *I'm sorry we've not had much time together.*

I explain again about Dad's accident and the new arrangements in case she does not remember.

Mum: *That time has passed.*

Again, what an accurate, wise statement! She is telling me to be present.

Monday 11 September 2006

Mum: *I want something different, Margaret.*
Me: *What do you want to be different, Mum?*

I am sure I know what she means but still want to check out all the possibilities and not make any assumptions, as she has recently experienced a major change in her life.

Mum: *I don't know.*
Me: *Do you want to go back to your old home?*
Mum: *No.*
Me: *Do you want to go back to your old room?*
Mum: *No.*
Me: *Do you want to be free?*
Mum: [Emphatically] *Yes!*

I imagine she wants to be free from the limitations of her physical body. 'Free' was the word she used with reference to her dreams, right at the beginning of our journey, and freedom has been an on-going, important theme for her. This is not surprising, as she described herself as having 'hobbled feet'. I can help her to find freedom through visualization and maybe by talking to her.

Mum: *I'm trying to find words. You're asleep.*
Me: *I'm asleep or I need to sleep?*
Mum: *You need to sleep.*

She is absolutely right. I am exhausted after all that has happened.

Tuesday 12 September 2006

Mum is struggling and Dad is struggling. The last thing he ever wanted was to end up in a care home with all these 'old people'. And here he is, the only resident who does not have dementia, a prisoner in an old people's home filled with old ladies in various stages of deterioration, and subject to the institution's many routines and constraints.

I considered arranging round-the-clock care for him in our house, but he would require two carers on duty for each of the three eight-hour shifts. It would be very difficult if he didn't like any of his carers. (On occasions in the past he has refused to allow certain carers cross his threshold!) I also know from experience that arrangements don't always work out as planned. Carers may not turn up because they are sick or the bus doesn't come or for some other valid reason, and it isn't always possible to find a substitute. If I were on hand the arrangement might just be feasible but I couldn't be on call all the time. Also the house isn't designed to cater for his current needs and would be hard to convert.

Mum: *What a down come.*

Reflections,
Revelations and
Recommendations

REFLECTIONS ON OUR JOURNEY

'We had a difficult beginning but we've had a good ending.'
Pat

Our earthly journey together has come to an end and it is time now to stop, to reflect and appreciate some of the extraordinary things that happened during our Heart and Soul Journey and along life's path: the dynamics that were operating in the family, the challenges each of us faced, the life choices we made and the transformations we went through.

My mother's experience when she had late-stage Alzheimer's was overwhelmingly positive and uplifting and she showed us the potential there can be in this advanced phase of the disease. She informed us in great detail about what she was experiencing in these last stages, of the disease. But perhaps more importantly, her Alzheimer's was a vehicle for teaching us all about the power of being present in the moment, the freedom that comes from releasing emotions, the healing power of love, the intricate and intelligent process of dying and the mysteries of the life beyond.

What was remarkable about my mother's experience was, first of all, the duration of her spiritual/end-of-life journey. Following her first initial deathbed vision of her demise, which is usually an indication that death is imminent, she continued to live for another three and a half years, during which she had a whole range of mystical experiences. The second remarkable factor was her ability to communicate what was happening to her, right to the end. This was exceptional – few people with Alzheimer's retain their faculty of speech and this degree of coherence in these later stages.

Considering for a moment the thoughts and feelings of those who have late-stage Alzheimer's and those observing them, it is important to note that it was only when my mother had moderate to severe Alzheimer's that she finally found peace and calm. This change from a negative state of mind to a positive one is reported in many people when they have reached this late stage and have surrendered to their condition. It suggests that much of the suffering that is talked about is in the eye of the beholder rather than in the person with Alzheimer's. If we acknowledge our own distress as a response to this situation, rather than projecting it on to our loved ones, maybe that will free us to engage with them in a more positive way.

I stated at the outset that my mother exhibited all the usual symptoms of Alzheimer's disease, including endless repetition and frequent confusion. But in the midst of all this there were many glimpses of wisdom, clarity and deep insight. These are what I retained and included in the journal entries about our Heart and Soul Journey, editing out most of the rest. This might have given the impression that my mother was different from other people, and readers could be forgiven for thinking I have romanticized her journey. But as you will discover, my mother was not alone in what happened to her. Others can have these positive experiences, too.

Our Journeys

The favourable circumstances of my mother's Alzheimer's without doubt facilitated our journey: the close proximity of the care home to our house, the quality of the care she received in the home, my availability and my skills and experience as a holistic therapist and healer. Not everyone will be so fortunate. I believe these optimal conditions enabled many extraordinary things to happen, and as a consequence we all have the opportunity to learn more about Alzheimer's disease, about the process of dying and about the Other World.

What happened to my mother and me was mutually beneficial – while I was supporting her, she was leading and teaching me. This symbiotic relationship enabled us to journey in ways I would never have imagined possible.

Mummy, it's me, Margaret.

I am with you.

You are going home. It will be wonderful.

Thank you for everything:
– For giving me life.
– For all you have taught me. It has changed me.

You are lovely, radiant.

You will be free. Free to move and dance.

We will always be together, united in spirit.

I love you.

And she slips peacefully into that Other World ...

Wednesday 17 January 2007

Dad is on the emergency operating list and I want to be with him, so I am at the hospital at 8.15am and stay there all day. What should have been a straightforward procedure turns out to be more complicated. I wait anxiously for hours, wondering what is happening and if he has died in the operating theatre. Surgery at his age and in his weakened state of health could easily be fatal. But he survives the operation and returns to the ward in a confused state having been given morphine. Not surprisingly, after this ordeal and being already exhausted, I fall ill with a sore throat.

Thursday 18 January 2007

There is no other family member around so even though I am not well I make brief visits to Mum in the care home and Dad in the hospital.

Sunday 21 January 2007

It is my birthday and I am laid up in bed with a sore throat and swollen glands. Because of this I have been unable to visit either Mum or Dad for the last couple of days.

Monday 22 January 2007

At 5.45pm I get a call from the care home. 'Your mum has had a turn. Come straightaway.' With my heart pounding, I get out of bed and rush next door. I know that this is it.

It is 6pm and Mum is in bed. Her colour is pale, almost opalescent, her eyes are closed, and her breathing is laboured. The staff nurse tells me she is dying. Now the meaning of Mum's puzzling remark, 'I didn't want to spoil, upset ... your birthday', spoken eighteen months ago, becomes clear to me. I phone a friend and try to arrange to get Dad discharged and back to the care home. He was going to be discharged tomorrow.

The Gift of Alzheimer's

I sit with Mum as she hovers between this world and the Other World, the world with which she has become so familiar. Her words come back to me, 'It's the climax. This is the end. It's peaceful.' With these thoughts in mind I have no fear. I hold her almost lifeless hand and kiss her gently, knowing that we are united in spirit. She seems unconscious, but I know that hearing is the last sense to go and that she may be able to hear me, so I behave as if she can. A deep stillness fills our sacred space as the veil between this life and the next dissolves and she floats toward that final moment of transition.

So, after a few hours organizing things, I am now on the train again heading back to Scotland, knowing that I am facing a difficult time on all fronts. I arrive home just before 10pm and go straight to the care home to see my parents, much as a mother checks her sleeping children before going to bed. First, I spend a few loving moments with Dad, who is sound asleep. Then I go upstairs to see Mum, who is also asleep. I kiss her ever so lightly and she opens her eyes and utters the word 'Amazing'. She looks absolutely radiant and beautiful and I notice that her breathing has speeded up momentarily with the excitement of seeing me. She then closes her eyes and goes back to sleep again. I will hold that magical moment in my heart and soul for ever.

Tuesday 16 January 2007

I spend the day at the hospital settling Dad in and going through all the preliminaries with the medical team. In the evening I visit Mum in the care home. She still has a bad cough and chest infection. I remember her words, 'I'm counting the months.' A lovely nurse who I know to be a devout Christian says to me, 'Tell your dad he's in my prayers. You're in my prayers, too. It must be hard for you having both parents not well.' Tears start to trickle down my cheeks and I look at Mum.

Me: [Apologetically] *It's all right to cry sometimes.*
Mum: *I don't bother.*

Well, my tears of self-pity instantly dissolve into tears of laughter. What a perfect antidote. She's done it again! She said exactly the right thing. How does she do it?

Mum: *Margaret is courageous.*

Interestingly, 'courageous' is the word that Paul used to describe me earlier in the day.

I talk about having an open heart.

Mum: *It's like floating.*
Me: *That's a beautiful description, Mum, and helpful to me.*
     Thank you.
Mum: [Emphatically] *You must tell William.*

So I note that my next mission is to help Dad to have an open heart.

Me: *I love you, Mum.*
Mum: *I know you do, Margaret. I see it in your eyes.*

This has been a most inspiring and uplifting evening.

2007

Monday 15 January 2007

I am in London, having reluctantly returned to teach the final module of my course, which was planned over a year ago. It is Monday morning and I am exhausted after seeing clients and then teaching for four consecutive days. My plan is to return to Scotland tomorrow after having today to catch up and recover. However, my phone rings and it is the hospital advising me that Dad is going in tomorrow for an emergency operation to remove the infected plate in his elbow. His health has been declining ever since his surgery last August, but despite this, and some very low moments, it is clear that he wants to go on living. As the infection was acquired in hospital I have pressed the consultant to take action and he has.

Mum: *Friends visit me.*
Me: *Who?*
Mum: *You.*
Paul is nice. He is intelligent.

We are very much in this reality just now. What she is saying about Paul is true. He is intelligent and intuitive and has a quiet manner. Mum recognizes and values these qualities.

Christmas Day 2006

After Mum has had Christmas lunch in the care home, Paul, Emily and I bring her round to the house for tea. She is quiet and struggles to cope, but with grace, as always. She is very weak now and can hardly sit and hold her head up, even with lots of support. After our family tea together I take her back to her other home next door, straining as usual to push the wheelchair over the chippings of our driveway. In the warmth of the care home, I settle her in and kiss her good night. As I walk back to our house on my own, in the cold and the dark, my heart is heavy. It is almost unbearable. I go straight to my room as I need to be quiet and on my own at this time.

Boxing Day 2006

Mum: *You're not departing?*
Me: *No I'm not. I'm very happy to be here with you for a while.*

Wednesday 27 December 2006

Mum: *You have a lovely smile.*
Me: *Thank you. Do you want me to talk to you or be quiet?*
Mum: *Talk to me.*

We talk and she says that Paul is very nice, just as she did a few days ago.

Mum: *You have done well.*
Me: *Thank you, Mum. So have you, very well.*
Mum: *You talk to me. Nobody else talks to me.*

Tears stream down my face as she says this. It is one of the saddest things she has said. It is so wonderful being with her but I am the only person who talks to her in a way that is meaningful to her and lets her know that I understand her. This journey started three and a half years ago as she was baring her soul and searching for the truth. I connected to her with an open heart and listened with an open mind and we talked. It was that simple.

Thursday 28 December 2006

Mum is in bed, bright-eyed and alert. Delightful.

Mum: *You have lovely teeth. You have a lovely complexion. You have lovely lips. Margaret has done well. I am happy at last.*

Well, despite everything, she hasn't lost her ability to observe me and tell me how lovely I am!

She is finally happy, because Margaret has done well. Was that her mission – to make up for what she hadn't been able to give me before? If so she has succeeded beyond anything I could have imagined in my wildest dreams. She is happy. I am happy. We are happy. We have overcome.

I notice that when she talks about my physical aspects she refers to me in the second person. However, when she refers to me in the third person, saying 'Margaret has done well', I believe she is talking to me on a non-physical plane.

I tell her about my daily practice of mindfulness meditation and healing prayer that takes me into a non-physical space. This practice, as well as benefiting me personally, has resulted in many miracles for others over the years.

Mum: *You must practise.*

to feel whatever is present. By doing this and not repressing my feelings, I will process them in my own time.

Me: [Feeling anxious as I ask her] *How many stages are there, Mum?*

Mum: *Seven.*

I wonder how long it will take for her to progress through these final seven stages, how many months. Her answer shows her awareness about the process of dying. She is accessing knowledge that comes from beyond our physical world. I wonder if the seven stages relate to the seven chakras or energy centres and the seven levels of the human energy field. Might this be a final process that involves moving through the different energetic levels to the highest energy or frequency in preparation for passing over?

Mum: *You have beautiful eyes. Margaret is happy.*

I am glad Margaret is happy but to be honest I am feeling a bit shaky.

I talk to Mum about my belief that death is not final but merely a transition from one form of being to another, as we move from one frequency in this world to a different one in the Other World. We are together now and we will continue to be together in spirit, wherever she is and I am. Her eyes are bright and searching as she listens eagerly to what I am saying. She is so frail I have to be careful not to overwhelm her with my robust energy.

My thoughts and beliefs come from a number of different sources, some spiritual and some scientific, as well as an intuitive sense of knowing.

Friday 22 December 2006

It will be Christmas in three days and I feel so relieved to be in Scotland for a few weeks.

Me: *Hello Mum. It's so lovely to see you. How are you? How are you feeling?*
Mum: *Average. It's lovely to see you, Margaret.*
Me: *Yes, we're making up for lost time.*

Mum is in bed and looking bright, despite a rattling cough that is persisting despite courses of antibiotics. I realize this could develop into pneumonia at any time and that that would be the end.

Christmas is a very busy time and I step back to give Paul and Emily, who aren't around so much, space to connect with their granny in their own ways. I am aware that this might be the last time they can do this.

Mum: *You're a good mother.*

She understands intuitively what I am doing. I don't need to explain anything to her any more.

Me: *Yes, and it's time now for me to be a good mother to you, too.*
          What are you thinking, Mum? You don't need to say anything if you don't want to.
Mum: *My thoughts are confused. It's progressive. I'm bored lying in bed.*
          Margaret hasn't lost anything. Margaret has found the secret.

This is so true. In our sacred space Mum has taken me to the Other World and brought the Other World to me. Through this I have 'found the secret' and feel blessed beyond belief. This is the ultimate gift, the gift of all gifts, and I thank her from the depths of my heart and soul.

Tuesday 14 November 2006

Me: *You look so young and lovely, Mum.*

She really does. She looks utterly radiant.

Mum: *I feel young.*
Me: *What age do you feel?*
Mum: *Seventeen – ten years older.*
Me: *Older than what?*
No reply.

No reply has always signified a connection with the Other World. Where is Mum now? When she was twenty-seven she was carrying me in her womb.

––––––––––––––––––––

Monday 27 November 2006

I have just arrived and Mum, who is sitting at the far end of the residents' lounge, is waving to me. She sees me before I see her.

Me: *Hello Mum. It's so lovely to see you again. How are you?*
Mum: *Fine.*
      [After a pause] *I have entered the first stage.*

Suddenly, I am struck by the reality of this: the end of her life is approaching – no more rehearsals. I feel empty and can hardly think. It is as if all the knowledge I have gained about death and the dying process has suddenly gone out the window. She is my mum and I love her so much. I am going to miss her terribly.

Reflecting on my feelings, I realize that my distress is due to my feelings of impending loss. Mum will be fine, I am absolutely sure about that. But how will I be? How will I cope with losing her? I reassure myself that my feelings are normal and that it is important that I go with the flow and allow myself

194

I imagine she is empathizing with me over the difficult circumstances.

Tuesday 31 October 2006

Mum: *We can't go on for ever. Things change.*
You're in the presence of kings and queens.

Another announcement, but this time it is different. Now she is telling me directly that she is going to die. It is hard for me to hear this.

I feel deeply moved and know I am very, very privileged to be 'in the presence of kings and queens'. This is indeed a sacred space right now. She said 'you', not 'Margaret', which suggests these energetic beings are with us, here, now. I imagine she is seeing or sensing the presence of entities of a very high vibration, possibly Masters and Archangels from the Angelic Kingdom. I am still and feel completely present.

Wednesday 1 November 2006

Dad: [To me] *I don't know what I would do without you.*
Mum: [To me] *I don't know what I would do without you.*

I am spending most of my time in the care home now.

Monday 13 November 2006

After a brief visit to London to teach the third module of my training course, I am back and very relieved to be here.

Me: *Hello Mum. It's lovely to see you. How are you?*
Mum: *I don't have anything to say.*
Me: *That's fine. There's no need. You've said so much.*

My mother's natural ability as a teacher enabled her to instruct me and to recognize the importance of what we were learning. My experience as a healer, teacher and writer enabled me to fulfil her wish to pass on this information to others so that they might benefit, too.

My Mother's Journey

My mother suffered from mental instability from the time I was born, but I am wondering now if the acute anxiety she experienced might have arisen from a feeling of slipping out of this world, much the same as she later experienced when she was suffering from Alzheimer's. This would have led to a sense of deep insecurity as she had adult responsibilities then and was trying to function normally in the world.

There was a stigma attached to mental illness in those days so people had to conceal their distress. Also, there was little understanding of my mother's kind of illness and there was no medical treatment for it. Not surprisingly, my father did not know what to do and he did not have the resources to support his wife emotionally.

As time went on my mother's distress was exacerbated by the social mores that severely limited the scope of women. She bore the cross of women trapped in this era and was a brave voice in conservative provincial Scotland.

When her physical and mental faculties atrophied due to Alzheimer's, she started to experience intermittent altered states of consciousness in which her inner senses awakened. This opened a channel to the Other World in which she had many extraordinary experiences. She frequently left her body and returned, she had contact with deceased relatives, she received instructions about the dying process and she previewed her own death and her life after death. These phenomena could so easily have been dismissed out of hand as delusional perceptions or hallucinations as experienced in mental illness.

During this time she also developed the gifts of extrasensory perception: telepathy, precognition, clairvoyance, clairaudience, clairsentience, mediumship and channelling, which she demonstrated quite naturally and unselfconsciously. She described seeing pictures and hearing sounds through her inner 'television' – her portal to the Other World. Although she was unaware of it, this is exactly how many psychics describe channelling information from the Other World.

The last few years of her life were, without doubt, very positive and this was the direct result of her having Alzheimer's. The disease enabled her to give and receive love as she had not done before and to have wonderful Other World experiences that prepared her for a good death and for her next journey.

Two Worlds

At the beginning of our journey my mother said, 'It's difficult being ... working between two worlds.' In this world she suffered all the common distressing symptoms of Alzheimer's, but in the Other World she was free in mind, body and spirit. The dynamics that were operating between us were also very different in each world. In this world I supported and held her, and at times led her. But in the Other World she spoke with a voice of absolute authority and led me.

Her exceptionally clear perception of everything, especially near the end, and her gift of extrasensory perception, were not of this world. She told me things about myself that came from the Other World and these were, without exception, 100 per cent correct. It was the accuracy of this personal information that validated her Other World for me and convinced me that the other things she was telling me were in fact true.

We only truly know something when we experience it ourselves, so I encourage others to be curious, find out for themselves and draw their own conclusions. Instead of dismissing the pronouncements of people with Alzheimer's as being purely delusional, I suggest that it would be wise to listen with an open mind to these voices from beyond the veil.

My Journey

This journey with my mother has changed my life. She said reassuringly, 'It will never leave you. It's part of you', and I can confirm this to be true.

There is a difference between believing and knowing. I started our journey believing, my beliefs based on what I had learned throughout my adult life as a seeker of consciousness. My mother just *knew*. Her knowing came directly to her from the Other World. As she taught and guided me on our journey, my believing changed to knowing. This was a profound change and a wonderful gift.

Like most people, I had no prior knowledge of Alzheimer's and once it started I didn't have time to stop and find anything out. This meant that throughout I was acting intuitively. My mother presented me with the perfect circumstances through which I could gain the experience I needed of Alzheimer's and the Other World, and *know*, not just know about.

My own quest as a seeker of consciousness may have arisen initially from my need to find deeper meaning, having experienced my early life as being so difficult. My sensitivity to energy I believe resulted from me having had to be hyper-vigilant as a child, because of the uncertainty and danger around my mother. As a consequence of my mother's difficulties during my childhood, I was later motivated to heal my past and was drawn to train in a number of healing modalities. At the end of my mother's life I was in a position to bring my knowledge and skills back to her and to help her. This demonstrates the ripple effects of a deeply healing process.

Through our journey I discovered the true meaning of compassion and unconditional love, and my heart was opened in a new and wonderful way. This led to profound healing and a reconciliation of our previously damaged relationship. The symbiosis that developed from our mutual love and appreciation was absolutely beautiful and filled me with joy and gratitude. It gladdened my heart and fed my soul and I can still feel the *lift* in my energy when I think of it now. My mother said to me near the end of her life, 'We had a difficult beginning but we've had a good ending.' Her remark sums up the story of our lives together and the amazing transformation that occurred.

The unexpected gift to me was her sojourns in the Other World. At the time I was only able to share the extraordinary experiences we were having with a very small number of people; I felt inhibited when family members or other people were around. Many of the things my mother said, when taken in isolation, were hard to comprehend, and only when considered as part of a whole did their meaning become clear. The Other World I am talking about is created of invisible energy and exists in sacred space. I came to understand the need for me to be in a quiet place in which I could be totally present when engaging in this dimension.

Reflecting on my behaviour toward my mother, prior to our journey, it is only now that I am realizing just how deep the wounds were from my childhood. There were times when I think I may have been very hard on her, more so than she deserved. I think I developed protective armour at an early age, and despite my many years of therapy this remained firmly in place until the start of our journey, when she was vulnerable and was no longer a threat. But I should not reproach myself; as I said to my mother, 'We make the best choices we can at the time.' I have mentioned the wise friend who told me that the positive things I was experiencing on our journey were 'payback' for me, but in truth it was payback time for my mother, too. I would say it was balanced, as it should be.

The re-opening of old wounds between my mother and me, between her and my father, and between other family members, has been very therapeutic for me. Before I started this journey I thought I had done 'the work', but clearly there still was more to do. Writing about our story has made me stop and think more deeply, and through this I have gained even greater insight and understanding that has resulted in a very deep personal healing. I am grateful to have had the opportunity to do this.

Reflecting on the very end of our journey, I ask myself now why I didn't just stay with my mother during her final weeks. The answer is this: having been through so many rehearsals for her death over the years, I imagined it would take many more months. I had long-standing commitments to my students that I felt obliged to honour. Had I known, when my mother said near the end, 'I have entered the first stage', that the seven stages she mentioned then were going to take only seven weeks, I would have cancelled my course and remained with her. In retrospect it seems an error of judgement on my part, but I was with her at the end as she had predicted – 'Margaret and I can be in the house together'.

The Lost Roses

The Lost Roses vignette is, in its fullness, symbolic of the experiences of my mother and I along the paths of our lives.

'The lost roses' is what my mother said to me as I was thinking about a card I had sent to her for Mother's Day.

There were twelve roses on the card. I had made it for her.

She never received it. The card was lost.

A rose is a flower of exquisite beauty and a symbol of love. The interweaving petals are like the many aspects of life. Together they form a perfect whole.

Its scent warms the heart and lifts the spirits. Its thorns protect the flower.

If you attempt to reach this expression of love, the thorns can cause hurt. But once you have reached the rose, its beauty and perfection fill your heart.

The roses card was my gift to my mother on Mother's Day.

This was to say thank you for the gifts she had given to me as my mother.

Not only for the gift of this life but for the ultimate gift, the gift of all gifts, the gift of life everlasting.

The card was lost.

This loss was symbolic, and a reminder of the losses in her life and mine and the loss we both experienced in relation to each other over a lifetime.

'The lost roses' was my mother's gift to me.

Unlike my gift, which was a symbol of this world and was lost, my mother's gift was not of this world.

Her words, 'The lost roses', showed me that although my card with its gift of love never arrived, she nevertheless knew about it and had received my message.

Healing Our Family Constellation

This journey did not only affect my mother and me. The most wonderful gift is that it had an impact on everyone in our family and through it we were all able to heal, including my sister Fiona who had already passed on.

My father's life presented him with extreme emotional challenges. Following his shocking experience at the age of eleven, when he discovered his own father lying dead on the floor, his way of dealing with emotions was to immediately cut himself off from them and move on quickly. My mother's volatile emotions challenged him constantly throughout his life and the more she confronted him, the more he tried to escape. He and my mother were at opposite ends of the emotional spectrum and remained locked in this polarized position for most of their lives.

At one point in our story, when my father was still living independently at home, but lurching from one crisis to another, he said to me, 'Give me a pill. I want to end it now!' Understandably, he feared what lay ahead, seeing nothing positive, nothing at all. But had he ended his life at this point, he would not have gone on to experience the resolution with my mother that was so important for both of them at the close of their lives. As my parents have demonstrated, people in the final stage of life, whose physical and mental faculties have greatly diminished, can enter a new phase in which they find love, peace and resolution. This demonstrates that it is never too late to seek redemption and heal the past.

My mother's mental instability and my father's emotional absence resulted in tensions and battles that impacted on my sister and me. Having a positive vision as a seeker may have motivated me to seek resolution through psychotherapy and spirituality. My sister may not have had such a vision or opportunity, and I surmise she sought to drown her childhood traumas in alcohol and as a result died prematurely.

However, although not physically present, my sister was a key player in the later evolution of our family and without her I would not be telling this story now. Anchored in this world I held the space for my mother to cross over into the Other World and return. There in the Other World she met her deceased daughter and afterwards told me, 'Everything, my ideas, thoughts are from Fiona. She's done it.' My mother acted as a channel for my sister to pass on information that over time healed all the members of our family and also fulfilled my deepest desire: to know about the Other World.

I realize now what a wonderful gift my sister gave to us all and what a price she paid. I feel humbled when I think about it. So I thank her from the depths of my heart and soul for the part she played in enabling all the members of our family to be healed in such an extraordinary way. It makes me wonder what we can ever really know about the mysteries of life and death. Who are we to judge others? What grand plan, of which we are unaware, is weaving its way through our daily lives right now?

My Parents' Shared Journey

What brought my mother and father together? Was it the attraction of opposites, the feminine and masculine, the yin and the yang? If so, the opposition may have been too strong. Both were extrovert individuals and I wonder if there just wasn't room for two such personalities to co-exist harmoniously.

Some of the seeds of the disharmony my parents experienced were sown during the war. They, like many couples of their era, married with little time to get to know each other. Life was very uncertain. When the men returned from the war, if they returned, they just had to get on with it. At the centre of the unhappiness at home was my mother's mental instability. Divorce was not really an option – it was deeply frowned upon. If this marriage had existed in a different era and a different environment, might it have had a different outcome? But my parents struggled, staying together but in many ways apart, until they were at the end of their lives. Then, in the frailty and vulnerability of old age, a new understanding and appreciation developed between them that turned out to be deeply healing.

Was there something else that kept their connection all those years? Searching to find an answer to this question I realized that throughout their lives they were both attracted, almost addicted, to the same colour: lovat blue, a soft turquoise. It was always their first choice for everything, from clothes to cars. Each colour has a frequency and this has an effect on our being. So at this vibrational level they were closely connected throughout their lives together.

Some mystics say turquoise is the colour associated with the lost civilization of Atlantis, a legendary island whose people are believed to have achieved an exceptionally high level of spiritual development. Pondering on this for a moment, and allowing myself to drift off into a wild fantasy, I wondered if my parents had shared past lives together in Atlantis, the lost turquoise island, and chosen to come together again in this life to learn and resolve some unfinished business ...

Returning to our all-important aspirations here in this world, is the transformation that my parents went through – this loosening of structures, beliefs and values – possible for everyone at the end of life? If the right conditions are in place, can we all find resolution and heal our past?

I believe we can.

THE OTHER WORLD AND THE
NEUROSCIENCE OF ALZHEIMER'S

'We are learning we're immortal.'
Pat

Contrary to popular expectation, what my mother and I experienced when she had late-stage Alzheimer's was exceptionally positive. This raised many questions. Was our experience unique? What broader conclusions could we draw from it? Could others enjoy something similar? Were there explanations for some of the things that happened?

In order to answer these questions I needed to look beyond our personal experience and this took me on yet another journey. One path led me to innovative research into the care of Alzheimer's, another to the field of neuroscience, and yet another to mystical teachings originating from the Other World. My findings from these disparate sources were for me no less than revelatory and led me to make some propositions, which I am putting forward here.

Emotional Memory

When my mother couldn't remember what she had just said, it would be easy to presume that she couldn't remember other things, too. However, she did remember some things very clearly. What could be the explanation for this?

In research on memory and ageing published in 2011, Professor Oliver Turnbull of Bangor University discovered that in Alzheimer's, despite episodic memory impairment, emotional memory is not lost – it seems to remain intact.[1] This could explain the distressing 'life reviews' my mother had, as well as some of the seemingly irrational emotional behaviour others with Alzheimer's exhibit from time to time. Carl Jung recognized this when he said about the end of life, 'Forgotten or repressed material surfaces in a state of diminished consciousness.' Turnbull found that people with Alzheimer's continue to learn from their emotional experiences and this could explain why positive feelings grew between my mother and me when her other functions were in decline.

Empathy and Emotional Contagion

When my mother had late-stage Alzheimer's, our relationship changed from having been quite challenging to being deeply loving. Was this kind of change exclusive to us?

Not according to scientific research led by Virginia Sturm at the Memory and Aging Center at the University of California, San Francisco, and published in 2013. Her work shows that as parts of the brain, particularly the temporal lobe, are destroyed by Alzheimer's disease and cognition decreases, the area of the brain that deals with empathy becomes more active. People become very sensitive to the feelings, expressions, words and behaviours of others. Surprisingly, as cognitive skills decline, empathy increases exponentially.

Furthermore, Sturm found that when people with Alzheimer's are empathetic and 'tuned in' to those around them, they respond by mirroring back what they are sensing. This unconscious ability to mimic is called 'emotional contagion'.[2] These findings highlight the fact that Alzheimer's sufferers are extremely vulnerable to the feelings of others, and this has *huge* implications for all those involved with people with Alzheimer's.

This research shows that the deeply loving relationship that developed between my mother and me is a real possibility for everyone.

Body, Mind and Soul Contagion

If neuroscientists have established that *emotional* contagion happens in people with Alzheimer's, it raises the question of whether contagion is happening at other levels too, such as those of the body, the mind and the soul. Speaking as an energy therapist and healer, I know contagion occurs at all these levels, even if it has not been described in these terms before. My mother demonstrated body contagion when she said, 'Your teeth, are they alright?' She demonstrated mind contagion when she referred to 'the lost roses', and soul contagion when she said, 'I can tell everything through the eyes'.

To what extent was contagion occurring between my mother and me at the mind and soul levels? Was I influencing her and was she influencing me? I think it is quite likely this mutual influencing was happening, however I don't believe it in any way invalidates what we experienced or my understanding of what my mother was trying to communicate.

If my mother experienced contagion at all these levels, then there is no reason to presume that other people with Alzheimer's don't or can't experience this, too. If we accept this hypothesis, then it may be that people with Alzheimer's are picking up much more from those around them than we previously thought. Food for thought!

Hard-wired for Love

When my mother had late-stage Alzheimer's, she time and time again expressed universal loving thoughts. 'I love everyone,' she said, and despite her severe disabilities she still had a deep, on-going need to care for me. According to John Zeisel, visiting professor at the University of Salford, Manchester, scientific advisor at the Salford Institute for Dementia and author of *I'm Still Here*, these kinds of thoughts and feelings are 'hard wired' into the human system and are therefore common to everyone, including those with Alzheimer's.[3] His research shows that people with Alzheimer's, whose thoughts are not censored in the way ours are, frequently express openly loving thoughts and feelings when they are given the right kind of support and validation.

The Power of Love

What is happening when unconditional love is present? In her 1997 book *Molecules of Emotion*,[4] neuroscientist Candace Pert explains that there is a biomolecular basis for emotion. Albert Einstein proved that when matter, such as molecules and atoms, is broken down into smaller components we move beyond the material realm into a realm in which everything is energy. Energy vibrates and the speed at which it vibrates is its frequency. Frequency is measured in hertz (Hz) – one vibrational cycle per second equals one hertz.

One doesn't need to be a physicist or a healer to know that the feeling of love is very different from the feeling of fear. Healers who can sense energy tell us that each emotion vibrates at a different frequency[5]: feeling love generates a faster vibration and higher frequency than feeling fear. This brings us to another important principle in physics, that of resonance. When two frequencies, such as those of the human body, are brought together, the lower one will *always* rise to meet the higher one. This explains why love will eventually triumph over adversity.

All religions and spiritual teachings tell us that love is the gateway to heaven or the Other World, and this implies that energetically speaking the invisible Other World has a faster vibration and higher frequency than our material world. My mother and I were both resonating at the frequency of love; through empathy she felt my love for her and through emotional contagion she reflected it back to me. I believe it was feeling love that enabled her, when she was in an altered state of consciousness, to access the Other World and have such positive experiences.

This raises the question of whether everyone with Alzheimer's, when they are in an altered state of consciousness, feeling love and resonating at this frequency, might be able to access the Other World and have positive experiences. I believe this is a real possibility. And when *we*, as family, carers or friends, of people with Alzheimer's, are resonating at this frequency, then we benefit, too. This is the power of love.

Conscious Dying

The dying process my mother went through was not unique. Eastern religions such as Hinduism and Buddhism, as well as shamanic traditions, provide explicit teachings that guide the dying to a conscious and graceful death. In the late sixties this practice was introduced to the West and became known as the conscious dying movement, pioneered by Cicely Saunders.[6] This treats death as an opportunity for both the dying and those close to them to become more present and more loving and to go through a profound healing and a spiritual awakening. Alzheimer's is a protracted end-of-life experience and this allows us more time to appreciate what is happening and to engage in the dying process with a greater level of consciousness.

Extraordinary End-of-Life Experiences

My mother had many extraordinary experiences when she had late-stage Alzheimer's. Were these unique to her? In their 2008 book *The Art of Dying*, Peter Fenwick and Elizabeth Fenwick give countless examples of deathbed visions, spontaneous states of euphoria, unexpected lucidity, extraordinary light, apparitions and much more.[7] These findings were drawn from Peter Fenwick's extensive research in the field and suggest that some people when they are dying enter an altered state of consciousness in which they have access to a different reality, one that is not normally available to us in everyday life. My mother experienced all the above phenomena, and others with Alzheimer's may have extraordinary experiences, too. Because these altered states of consciousness happen over an extended

221

period of time in Alzheimer's, not just at the very end of life, we have the possibility of 'tuning in' and sharing in the wonder of this other dimension, the Other World.

Near-death Experiences

When people come back to life after having been declared clinically dead, they are said to have had a near-death experience (NDE) or a transitory death experience (TDE). Following such an event many people have a spiritual awakening that dramatically changes their lives. According to Raymond Moody, they no longer fear death, they become more loving, their values change and they become less materialistic.[8] I observed some of these changes in my mother and now I wonder if she, too, had a near-death experience, an undetected one.

About nine months before I started to record our Heart and Soul Journey, as I mention in my introduction to that part of the book, my mother was found deeply unconscious by the care-home night staff. Initially they failed to get any response from her, but she eventually came round and miraculously seemed none the worse for this medical emergency. She did not talk about her experience to me at the time, but reflecting on what happened subsequently I wonder if she had an NDE when she was unconscious. If this happened to her, might others with Alzheimer's or who are approaching the end of life also have undetected NDEs that result in them having a spiritual awakening?

Consciousness

The location of consciousness is one of the biggest unsolved mysteries of all time and continues to give rise to fierce debate. In the Western medical world consciousness is understood to be a function of the brain. However, not everyone agrees with this view. Rupert Sheldrake, a distinguished and controversial biologist, fellow of the Institute of Noetic Sciences in California and previously a fellow at Cambridge University, hypothesizes the existence of 'extended mind' in which consciousness, or mind, exists outside as well as inside the brain.[9] The view of consciousness existing outside the brain is substantiated by many of those who have had an NDE. According to a 1975 work by Raymond Moody, many people who are declared clinically dead, during which time their brain 'flatlines' (shows no electrical activity) later describe having been out of their body.[10] They frequently recount, among other things, looking down from above at what is happening below and report what they see and hear in great detail, including what is happening to their own body and what people are saying about it. These accounts are generally verified as being totally accurate.

Consciousness is defined as 'a person's awareness or perception of something'.[11] So if people have awareness and perception when they have no brain activity during an NDE, this suggests that their consciousness, at that time, was not a function of their brain. Similarly, people with Alzheimer's and others at the end of life, when their cognitive function has severely declined, can still have acute awareness and perception. This again suggests that consciousness is not entirely a function of the brain.

Researchers such as Lynne McTaggart (2001[12]) and Ervin László (2004[13]) describe consciousness as a *universal* field of information. Viewed from this perspective the individual brain becomes the receiver for and transmitter of information to and from the universal field. If we think of information as a continuum of frequencies, then the specific frequency we are tuned in to will be determined by our state of consciousness at the time. An analogy would be turning on the radio: we select a wave band, tune in to a frequency and listen to the information that is coming through on that frequency. Viewing consciousness in general in this way would accommodate different states of consciousness, including those experienced by people with Alzheimer's, in this and the Other World.

Transcendence

In Alzheimer's disease the brain slowly disintegrates, causing a gradual breakdown in physical and mental capabilities. This results in the dissolution of the self – the loss of the personality and the ego. The sufferer's perception of time also changes. Time is no longer experienced as linear – past and future move into the present and there is only the 'now'. Being totally present in the 'now', and at the same time having no ego, is being in a transcendental state. This is the state seekers of consciousness are aiming to find. It is what Eckhart Tolle teaches in his seminal book *The Power of Now* (1999).[14] I believe it is being in a transcendental state that enables people with Alzheimer's to experience other levels of consciousness.

Other Worlds and Parallel Universes

My mother said, 'It's difficult being ... working between two worlds.' One world she described was our physical world in which she had all the common losses and limitations of Alzheimer's. However, she also talked about another world, a world in which she was completely at peace, free from worry and fear, and in which she felt universal love for everyone. So she did indeed experience two worlds and each was distinctly different.

The suggestion that we might exist in two or more worlds simultaneously is not just a mystical or religious one; it has a scientific basis. In 1933 the eminent physicist Sir Oliver Lodge FRS put forward the proposition that at the micro level there are two worlds: the atoms, of which matter is made, and the energy field, the seemingly empty space that surrounds and drives them.[15]

In the 1950s another eminent physicist, Hugh Everett, put forward the hypothesis of many worlds, and today the multiverse and parallel universes (the various universes within the multiverse) are at the forefront of scientific enquiry. The multiverse hypothesis is supported by many of the world's leading quantum physicists, including Stephen Hawking. Work like Brian Greene's 2011 book *The Hidden Reality* posits that according to mathematical calculations we may actually exist in more than one world at the same time.[16]

Although we can't prove that there is more than one world, we can't disprove it, either, and I would suggest that like the physicists we keep an open mind. When people are in an altered state of consciousness, as they sometimes are in late-stage Alzheimer's, I believe that they are accessing another dimension and that the information or frequency in their field at that time will determine which Other World they enter.

Revelations of the Other World

Throughout the last three and a half years of her life, my mother described her progress through various phases and stages that demonstrated to me that dying can be an intelligent process. Searching to find out more about this, I was amazed to discover that the stages of dying she discussed with me are the same, and occurred in the same order, as those described by a spirit entity, Michael, to a medium in this world, Victoria Marina-Tompkins.[17] There is one difference, however: my mother had these experiences while she was here in the physical realm, whereas the entity tells us that these same phases occur in the Other World during the inter-life – the period *after* death and before the next life.

Near the end of her life my mother referred to entering the first of a further set of seven stages, which seemed to be associated with the very close of the dying process. She and I had never discussed seven stages of dying and this concept had certainly had not been part of her Presbyterian background, so where did this information come from? As Helena Blavatsky pointed out back in 1880, the number seven has been considered sacred throughout antiquity and has had significance in all major cultures and religions.[18] This suggests to me that my mother was tuned in to sacred knowledge that was coming directly from another realm.

Does Alzheimer's in the later stages enable direct access to the Other World, access that is not normally available to us? I am proposing that it is the perfect vehicle for doing this. If we accept this hypothesis we might find that people with Alzheimer's can bring the Other World to us and teach us. But are we ready to listen and learn?

A Good Death

The research findings in this chapter confirm that the positive experiences my mother and I had when she had late-stage Alzheimer's were not unique to us but are a real possibility for others. So it seems that many people could meet death in a way that is similar to the wonderful approach of my mother. But for this to happen we need to listen for the wisdom in the midst of seeming incoherence, have an open mind as to what the person is saying, validate the person, and do all this with unconditional love. As our story shows, when we do these things love grows and the window to the Other World can open and reveal the hidden mysteries to us.

My conclusion is that Alzheimer's, being a protracted end-of-life experience, in which people have altered states of consciousness and experience another reality, is the perfect vehicle for preparing for death and the Other World and can offer a wonderful process when love is present.

A POSITIVE WAY FORWARD:
CARE WITH KNOWLEDGE
AND UNDERSTANDING

'It's precious, Margaret, and should not be ignored.
You can tell others.'

Pat

It is time now to apply what we have learned to the care of people with Alzheimer's. Offering new insights and innovative approaches, along with a range of useful information, this chapter will serve as a comprehensive guide for family members, health-care professionals and educators. It pulls together what I learned on our Heart and Soul Journey, with research in the field and information from medical and non-medical experts and Alzheimer's organizations. Applying this knowledge and understanding to Alzheimer's care will bring about the best possible outcome for everyone and will help the realization of some of the hitherto hidden gifts of Alzheimer's.

(*Note*: The background to some of the information given in this chapter is provided in the previous chapter.)

Facts About Alzheimer's

What is Alzheimer's?

As stated in the Introduction, Alzheimer's is the most common type of dementia, accounting for 60 to 80 per cent of dementia cases. It is important, however, that a correct diagnosis is given as there are many different kinds of dementias, presenting in very different ways. Alzheimer's is a neurodegenerative disorder causing damage to parts of the brain that results in a plethora of neurological and physical disabilities. The disease is progressive and can take anything from five to twenty years before finally claiming the lives of those affected.

Symptoms of Alzheimer's

Symptoms vary according to the stage of the disease and from person to person. However, the following symptoms are common to all Alzheimer's sufferers at some stage: forgetfulness, anxiety, inability to manage complex life tasks such as dressing and toileting, immobility, rigidity and loss or partial loss of speech. Brain function slows down. People lose their sense of linear time and experience a diminished sense of self and a loss of identity.

Seven Stages of Alzheimer's

Descriptions of the seven stages of Alzheimer's make depressing reading, but it is important to identify which stage someone is currently at in order to understand what is happening to them and provide the most appropriate care and manage expectations. The Global Deterioration Scale (seven stages)[19] given here is widely used in diagnosis. As Alzheimer's is a progressive neurological disease the symptoms are many and varied. The duration of the seven stages can be seven years or more but not everyone will survive to the final stage.

Stage 1: Normal
As the term suggests this is the stage before the appearance of symptoms.

Stage 2: Normal aged forgetfulness
This is experienced by most people over the age of sixty-five. It can involve forgetting names and where they have left things, as well as difficulty in finding the right word when speaking.

I didn't tell her this. How did she know? She clearly has the ability to tune in to what is happening, even when it has slipped my mind. This is her eighth psychic reading of me.

Evening. Mum is in bed and I am lying down with her, giving her a loving hug.

Mum: *This is how Margaret wanted it. Margaret is nice. I will go to bed with Margaret hugging me.*

How lovely. What more could anyone want than the person they love most hugging them as they go to sleep? If only everyone could have this at the end of their life.

So she knows what Margaret wanted and what Margaret and I are going to do.

Me: *What are you thinking?*
Mum: *I don't have thoughts. My vocabulary is very scarce.*

This shows her level of awareness about her own condition. But it may be that in her current state, so near to the end of her life here in this world, and so close to the Other World, she has full awareness without having thoughts or words as such. She just knows.

Friday 27 October 2006

Mum and Dad are both unwell. Mum has a nasty rattling cough and Dad is getting weaker every day from an MRSA infection he acquired during the operation on his broken elbow. He wants to end it all. I am visiting Mum and Dad separately and trying to support them both.

Mum: *It's a shame about Margaret.*
Me: *What is a shame?*
Mum: *I don't know.*

Me: *We both know that death of the physical body is not the*
        end. When you leave your body you're still you in another
        world. You're free and can move and dance. You can
        practise leaving your body and coming back. You're free
        to choose, Mum.

I am talking about the Other World in the present tense, and also
using the words she has emphasized – 'free' and 'choose' – as
they are very relevant to this current transitional phase.

    I am sitting beside her, holding her fragile hand between
both my hands.

Mum: *This is doing me the world of good.*

Wednesday 25 October 2006

Afternoon. I have just arrived from London, after being there
briefly to teach the second module of my training course.

Mum: *Hello Margaret!*

Mum leans forward in her chair, having recognized me instantly
from where she is sitting on the other side of the large lounge.
I am so relieved. Whenever I haven't seen her for a few weeks I
fear that she may have deteriorated and might not recognize me
or might have lost her ability to speak.

Me: *Hello Mum. It's lovely to see you. How are you? How are*
        you feeling?
Mum: *Fine.*
        I want to be at all the meetings.

What meetings? I can't think what she is referring to. Then
I realize that one of my reasons for being here today is to attend
a meeting to formalize Dad's care arrangements in the home.

191

GOING HOME

'You're in the presence of kings and queens.'
Pat

Wednesday 4 October 2006

I have just arrived from London and I find Mum in her room, sitting in a chair by the bay window, with the patchwork blanket she knitted for me many years ago draped over her desperately thin legs.

Me: *Hello Mum, it's lovely to see you again. How are you?*
       How are you feeling?
Mum: *Fine.*
       I think we've done very well.
Me: *Yes, you're right, we have.*
Mum: *I'm counting the months.*

She is very lucid and clear and there is a sense of finality about what she is telling me – it sounds different from her previous comments about dying. My heart sinks. Throughout our journey she has demonstrated knowledge about her process of dying, so I believe she is giving me advance notice of her death in order to prepare me. After three years of rehearsals I had almost come to think it was never going to happen but I need to prepare myself now for the end. This is difficult, very difficult.

Thursday 5 October 2006

I want to talk more to her about death following her announcement yesterday.

190

Correct. Yet again she has found the perfect words to describe the situation. I am noticing that Mum's perception is getting clearer and clearer. I have to remind myself that she was officially diagnosed as having Alzheimer's disease in 2000, six years ago now.

Me: *I know you see things as they really are.*
Mum: *Yes.*
Me: *Although you can't always find the words, you still perceive the truth. You perceive everything as it really is.*
Mum: [Emphatically] *Yes.*

I would say, having faced her demons from the past, found redemption and forgiveness, and the capacity to love everyone, Mum has fulfilled all the core conditions for life's spiritual journey.

Me: *You're wonderful, Mum, really wonderful.*
Mum: *That's because I'm loved, Margaret.*

This is straight from the heart. I need to stop and take it in.

Me: *You've been a great help to me.*
Mum: *You're a lovely person.*
Me: *So are you, too lovely to put into words, Mum.*
Mum: *Where will you be next week?*

After our little exchange of mutual appreciation she is still able to think about the immediate future and knows I will not be here, although I haven't mentioned this to her.

Me: *I'll be in London.*
Mum: *There are so many things to remember. They're next door in the next room.*

Is this a metaphor for where she stores her memories?

Me: *What things?*
Mum: *I don't know.*

Wednesday 10 August 2005

Afternoon. I take Mum to her room. She is not always initiating conversations as she did in the past so I take this opportunity to reminisce with her about her teaching career. We talk about the time when she was a student at Dunfermline College of Physical Education in the 1930s, through her years of teaching in different schools, up to her retirement in 1975. She enjoys recalling these memories.

Mum: *You've helped me.*
Me: *You've helped me. We're helping each other.*

Mum: *After a long separation there is no need for words.*

I have been here for a week so we haven't had a long separation. Is she in a different timeframe, in the Other World?

Mum: *I am thinking of all the ways of thinking. I can't remember.*

She said back in December last year: 'I know my thoughts are clear. I'm confused when I can't remember.' But she is now saying she can't remember all the ways of thinking. She knows her memory is failing and she is trying so hard to find new ways in which she can continue communicating with me. I find this very touching.

Me: *Are you happy for me to ask you questions, Mum?*
Mum: *Oh yes, Margaret! Please do.*

She is moving her head from side to side as she does when she is silently processing thoughts. For the first time I decide not to wait until she has finished this routine sequence of movements, but instead to interrupt her mid-stream and try to catch her fleeting thoughts before they evaporate into the ether. I try this and it works – she is able to tell me what she is thinking. So this is the strategy I now need to employ in order to continue our communication.

Monday 8 August 2005

Evening. We are in Mum's room, having a joyous time. I am playing her favourite music and dancing around the room, trying to be graceful. She loves it. I wouldn't do this in front of anyone else and, as usual, pray a care assistant doesn't come in before I have had time to compose myself. The many secrets of Room 14!

Tuesday 9 August 2005

Mum is in her room.

151

now operating mainly through her energy body, she will manifest her thoughts quickly and effectively.

Evening. Mum is in bed.

Me: *When you're thinking, do you see pictures?*
Mum: *No, I hear voices.*
Me: *What kind of voices?*
Mum: *I don't know.*

I want to pursue this but she has moved on again to the enigma of Margaret and me.

Mum: *Margaret and you are meant to be different. That's just the way it is.*

So let it be. I place my hands on her to let the energy flow. She always feels this and likes it.

Sunday 7 August 2005

Morning. We have a short wheelchair walk then go to the garden at our house and sit in the sun for a while. Mum is wearing a floppy sun hat I got for her. It suits her perfectly.

Evening.

Mum: *I'm going home. I'm journeying.*
Me: *Are you with anyone?*
Mum: *Gillian.* [She doesn't know anyone called Gillian.] *I will come back next year.*
       I have lots of thoughts – they are jumbled up.

Her answers don't mean anything to me, so maybe they are jumbled-up thoughts. This is to be expected sometimes. Or maybe she is dipping into another reality. Who knows?!

information in a non-physical dimension. I really do find this gift of hers amazing and all the more so because she doesn't know she has it.

Mum: *I'm thinking a lot. How to say goodbye? How can I leave at night? I don't know. I need something at night.*

This is another reminder to me about her leaving. She has talked about 'night' before. I wonder what she is thinking.

Me: *What do you need?*
Mum: *Company? I don't know.*

I feel sad, as I would like to keep her company at night, but it isn't practical. I have to think of another way to comfort her.

Me: *You can be with angels and special friends at night.*
Mum: *What do they say?*
Me: *I don't know. They're always present. You just need to become aware of them.*
Mum: *I'm very happy. We're benefiting from having this time together.*
Me: *Yes, Mum, we are.*
Mum: *I'm getting better. It's wonderful.*

At the level of spirit she *is* getting better and it is wonderful.

Thursday 4 August 2005

Morning.

Mum: *I don't need to have company all the time.*

Oops! Maybe, following my suggestion, Mum asked for company and got more than she bargained for! 'Energy flows where attention goes'; this is how we manifest our thoughts. As Mum is

Stage 3: Mild cognitive impairment
The changes at this stage are subtle. People may repeat queries and have difficulty in mastering new skills and organizing things they could have done in the past. This can lead to increased anxiety.

Stage 4: Mild Alzheimer's disease
Difficulties at this stage are more pronounced, making diagnosis easier. People have decreased ability in managing complex daily tasks, such as arranging finances and planning and preparing meals, sometimes in writing the correct date. Practical help and understanding are needed at this stage. Duration: approximately two years.

Stage 5: Moderate Alzheimer's disease
At this stage people are at risk so are no longer able to live independently. They are more forgetful. They need assistance in choosing what to wear, paying bills, getting adequate food, etc. They are vulnerable to predators. Practical help and understanding of the issues, including emotional ones, are again needed. Duration: approximately eighteen months.

Stage 6: Moderately severe Alzheimer's disease
At Stage 6 professional help is required and this may be better provided in a care home. Stage 6 has five substages (total duration: approximately thirty-six months):

a. Assistance required in choosing clothes and getting dressed.
b. Inability to assess correctly the temperature of bath water and bathe themselves.
c. Assistance required in toileting and general hygiene.
d. Double incontinence. Little awareness of current address or the weather.
e. Difficulty in recognizing family members correctly and frequent confusion of spouse with someone else.

Stage 7: Severe Alzheimer's disease
Many people do not survive to this stage but if they do they require professional twenty-four-hour care. There are six substages. The most pronounced changes are neurological and these manifest in many ways, particularly in loss of muscle control and increasing rigidity.

    a. Speech is greatly reduced, to around half a dozen words.
       Duration: approximately one year.
    b. Speech is further compromised, to one word or sometimes nothing.
       Duration: approximately eighteen months.
    c. People are unable to move around independently.
       Duration: approximately one year.
    d. People are unable to support themselves when sitting. They also lose the ability to smile.
       Duration: approximately one year.
    e. Rigidity in facial expressions causes people to appear to grimace.
       Duration: approximately eighteen months.
    f. Vulnerable to pneumonia. Lose neck control and are unable to support the head.
       Duration: indeterminate.

Help for Alzheimer's: Core Care Conditions

There are certain core conditions that should underpin all aspects of Alzheimer's care.

Wellbeing

It goes without saying that creating a feeling of wellbeing is a core requirement for anyone who has Alzheimer's. Many relatives give excellent care at home and struggle on as the disease progresses, reluctant to abandon their loved one to a care home. However, there comes a time when a care home may be the best choice for the wellbeing of *all* concerned. A good residential home can provide the professional services required, a safe environment and, hopefully, compassionate and loving care. Having this in place enables family members to once again look after their own needs and frees them to engage in new ways with their loved ones.

Connection

Connection is at the heart of any good relationship and is especially important for people who have Alzheimer's. It isn't just *what* we say but, more importantly, *how* we communicate what we are feeling that matters. This is expressed through our eyes, tone of voice and facial expressions.[20]

People with Alzheimer's lose their inhibitions and can be very direct and demonstrative. In order for us to connect with them in a way that they understand, we sometimes need to step out of our comfort zone and join them in their world. This is likely to require us to be flexible in what we do and how we do it. Here are some basic guidelines for connecting with people with Alzheimer's:

- Sit at the same level as them.
- Look at them.
- Stop! Be aware of what you are feeling.
- If you are feeling compassion, let your heart open.
- Tell them you love them and care for them deeply (if you are feeling it).
- Give them 100 per cent of your attention.
- Smile and squeeze their hand, or whatever is appropriate, so that they feel your caring touch.
- If they can still talk, gently and sensitively ask them questions about themselves. Explain that you want to

231

know what they are feeling and thinking. Tell them it is all right if they don't answer.

- If they cannot speak, there are other ways to connect with them. They will sense and know what you are trying to communicate, and their heart will speak to you through their eyes. These can be the most precious, healing moments of all. Family members are important to people with Alzheimer's so do not mistake any lack of recognition for indifference. At the heart level the bonds remain forever strong.

Carl Rogers, founder of Humanistic Psychology and the Person-centred Approach, provided guidelines on how to relate that are helpful for everyone. Although he was referring primarily to the therapeutic relationship, he believed that the same principles apply to all human relationships. He said it is the *quality* of a relationship that really matters and concluded that at least three conditions are necessary[21]:

- Unconditional positive regard: always see the best in the person.
- Empathic understanding: listen with complete attention and with all your senses.
- Congruence: be authentic, real and honest. Be true to yourself.

Presence

In any relationship, being totally present when we are with the other person is what enables real connection, and this is particularly important with someone who has Alzheimer's. When we are present the person with Alzheimer's will be present with us. In fact, due to changes in the brain that slow everything down, they may be more in the moment, more present than we are.

Compassion and Love

Compassion is a response to witnessing another person's suffering and requires empathy. So witnessing the suffering of someone with Alzheimer's naturally gives rise to feelings of compassion. When we feel compassion it opens our hearts to love, and love is what someone with Alzheimer's needs most, not just to receive but also to give. Love can be expressed in many ways: verbally and non-verbally including gentle touch.

A Trusted Companion

When someone has lost control and can no longer manage life, what that person needs is a trusted companion. This was advocated by Naomi Feil, the founder of Validation Therapy.[22] Ideally, a companion should already know the person and be able to relate sympathetically to their personal circumstances and history. The companion does not have to be a professional. Being present, connecting with an open heart, listening with an open mind and responding sympathetically and without judgement is all that is required.

Validation

Feil recognized the need for validation for people with Alzheimer's and was a pioneer in promoting this. Sometimes giving validation is straightforward but at other times, when people say things that we don't agree with, it can be difficult. However, it is important to remember that what a person with Alzheimer's is experiencing is real for him or her. We can validate the person's experience without compromising our own position by the thoughtful use of language such as, 'That seems a very special ... for you' – and mean it.

Communicating with People with Alzheimer's

Our connection with others happens through communication and good communication is central to any relationship, especially relationships with people with Alzheimer's. But how can we connect with someone who isn't communicating clearly with us? It can be like trying to talk to someone in a foreign language that we don't understand. This section on communication aims to help to translate this 'foreign language' and bring greater understanding to what is happening during such communications.

Meaningful Communication

My mother said, 'You talk to me. Nobody else talks to me.' Of course other people talked to her, but no one talked to her in a way that was *meaningful* to her and let her know that she was understood. Dame Cicely Saunders, the pioneer in the UK of the hospice movement and the conscious dying movement, reported that she once asked a man who knew he was dying what he needed above all in those who were caring for him. His reply was simple: he wanted them to look as if they were trying to understand him.[23]

Meaningful communication is paramount in the care of Alzheimer's. How can we communicate meaningfully with people who have Alzheimer's when we don't understand what they are saying or doing? To know what they are thinking and feeling, we need to be flexible and move onto their map, travel with them in their world and respond from that position, rather than trying to impose our rational views on them. When we do this we will find ourselves entering into a new world, one that is wonderfully creative and full of the unexpected. Are you game for such an adventure?

Non-verbal Communication

Non-verbal communication is more important than verbal communication for people with Alzheimer's. It includes: facial expression (particularly the eyes); voice tone, speed and volume; touch and gesture. All these communicate what we are feeling, and feelings are what matter most. So being more aware of our non-verbal communication is more effective for reaching people with Alzheimer's than what we say and will enable a deeper and more meaningful connection.

Empathy

The ability to tune in to and understand another person's feelings is an important aspect of any relationship. However, empathy has particular importance when communicating with people with Alzheimer's because, as discussed above (see page 218), they develop a greater capacity for empathy as their cognitive skills decline and this increases exponentially as the disease progresses. This means people with Alzheimer's become ever more sensitive to nuances of expression and the feelings of others and will, if they can, communicate what they are sensing very directly to us. We may feel embarrassed by this as we are not accustomed to hearing such emotional honesty, but we can learn to accept it gracefully.

As we have seen, when people with Alzheimer's experience empathy and sense what we are feeling, they mirror our feelings back to us – they mimic us. This is what Virginia Sturm describes as 'emotional contagion' (see page 218). It happens verbally and non-verbally, and as a result a symbiotic relationship develops. Since we have more conscious control than they have, the emotional tone of the relationship is determined to a large extent by us. This places a huge responsibility on us and, hopefully, we can feel love and compassion in our hearts and be positive. However, we must be honest about our feelings, as the person will know what we are feeling even if we don't say it.

Touch

People with Alzheimer's can benefit enormously from touch, whether that's a gentle pat of reassurance on the arm or a full foot or hand massage. Touch promotes oxytocin, a neurotransmitter that brings about feelings of wellbeing,[24] so it can really help the person to relax.

Note: Always ask permission before doing any kind of massage and tell the person that they can say or indicate 'stop' at any time. When engaged in therapeutic touch, monitor the person's responses and if in any doubt check with them about how they are feeling.

Verbal Communication

Verbal communication is notoriously difficult with people who have Alzheimer's. Often they say things that make no sense to us, leaving us not knowing how to reply, let alone reply meaningfully. When they can't find the word they want to use, they may substitute a word that has the same or a similar meaning but is usually used in a different context, so we are none the wiser.[25] Thinking about the meanings and associations of any confusing word will give us a clue as to what they want to communicate.

People with Alzheimer's often use metaphor and this is rich in meaning. My mother said, 'Margaret left with something in her ear last night.' When I asked her what she meant, she said, 'The things I told her.' Talking about residents going to their rooms in the evening, my mother said, 'It's elastic.' The word she was looking for was probably 'flexible', but as she couldn't find it she used a word that does the same thing in another context. So be curious and explore their poetic world with them. Open a dialogue. Ask them questions, gently.

Distant Communication

It is not possible to be with our loved ones all the time. Although no substitute for being there in person, talking on the telephone is a way of keeping in touch if they can still speak. It is important when on the telephone to remember to express feelings through tone of voice, as well as verbally.

Directness

As a result of damage to the brain, people with Alzheimer's are very direct in their communication – they tell us exactly what they are thinking and feeling. The filters that we employ to temper our thoughts so that what we say is socially acceptable no longer work in people with Alzheimer's. This can result in them saying very positive things to us – or in the opposite. So be warned, you will hear the truth. Listen and respond with understanding.

Still Thinking

It is easy to assume, when people can't remember what they have just said or are unable to speak, that they are not able to think. I question this assumption because of what my mother told me. She made a distinction between thoughts and memory. She said, 'I know my thoughts are clear, I'm confused when I can't remember.' Toward the end of her life, when she was not so vocal and not volunteering information, I often asked her what she was thinking and my question prompted her to tell me. So I suggest that we keep an open mind about what they are thinking. We can ask them and should be prepared to be surprised at the response we get.

Keeping the Window Open

In the advanced stages of Alzheimer's, we can continue gently to ask questions like 'What are you thinking?' and 'What are you feeling?' This can sometimes stimulate them to engage with us if they can and want to, and it lets them know that we are still interested in them. It is also good to ask questions like 'Are you in any pain?' or 'Is there anything you need?' and monitor the response. Things change and information may not be volunteered unless the person is asked.

Subtle Energy Communication

Most people are unaware of the subtle energy that pervades and surrounds the physical body, but people with Alzheimer's, when they are frail, may be more sensitive to it. As the American physicist and spiritual healer Barbara Brennan pointed out in her 1987 book, *Hands of Light*, connecting with the energy field of another human being with love and light changes the energy of that field and the person feels the benefit of this physically and emotionally.[26] Even when someone cannot talk they may still benefit from this kind of healing energy connection. You don't need to be a 'healer' to do this. Just stop and become still, centre yourself and imagine the person bathed in a sea of love and light for a moment or two. Try it! You will discover how relaxing it is for you, too.

Understanding Memory and Emotions

Memories and emotions are intrinsically connected and this is the case in people with Alzheimer's, even when some of their memory is impaired. Knowing about this connection can help us to understand better what is happening to them and so improve the quality of their lives.

Memory

Short-term memory is processed in the brain by the hippocampus. This is where new information is filed. When this system isn't working properly, as in Alzheimer's, incoming information is sometimes incorrectly filed and therefore cannot be easily retrieved. However, those who seem to have lost their short-term memory can usually still access their long-term memory. We can help them to feel connected to their lives now by looking at and talking about things from the past, especially things that have particular meaning for them. Knowing they can still remember some things is very reassuring for people with short-term memory loss.

We have already seen (page 217) that not only does emotional memory seem to remain intact in people with Alzheimer's, but also that they can continue to learn from their emotional experiences right to the end of their lives. It is therefore helpful to revisit things from their past about which people with Alzheimer's have emotional feelings and attachments, such as people, pets, places, photos, songs and poems.

Changing Emotional Landscape

Feelings are paramount in Alzheimer's, however the type of emotions expressed will differ from person to person and will change at each stage of the disease.

In the earlier stages, feelings of anger are likely to arise from the internal struggle that occurs when people are losing their memory and ability to cope, but are still desperately trying to maintain some degree of control in their lives. This can be a very difficult time for carers.

As the disease progresses and people lose their memory and sense of identity they enter a new phase in which the mental structures that had once supported them cease to function effectively. This sounds a very unfamiliar and frightening place in which to find oneself. What do people experience in this phase?

Nature abhors a vacuum so something is going to fill it. But what kinds of feelings are going to flood into this gap: repressed painful memories from the past, random thoughts that just pop up out of nowhere and float by, good feelings, bad feelings? The retention of emotional memory could explain some of the unexpected and disturbing behaviour that some people with Alzheimer's exhibit. I suggest that we listen and try to help people to acknowledge their feelings so that their past can be healed.

Healing the Past

When difficult emotional memories surface, what should we do? Move on quickly to something else or listen and acknowledge what is being said or expressed? I believe the latter is what is needed and this is when the role of a trusted companion becomes all-important – someone to listen and bear witness as the person unburdens him or herself and seeks redemption. A helpful approach is to employ a presupposition of the sort used in Neuro-Linguistic Programming (NLP). You can tell the person, 'You did the best you could at the time – if you could have done anything better you would have done.' If you think about it, it is true. It is easy in retrospect to say you should have said or done something different, but at the time you did not have the knowledge or resources to do that. Acceptance of this kind can of course be applied to anyone, including oneself. When this affirmation is given with genuine love and understanding, it is often all that is required to release the person from their old feelings of guilt or shame. It can be followed up by talking about a more positive way forward. Once old emotional issues have been cleared and healed, the person is free from their burden and can move on and experience good feelings.

Impact of Changes to the Brain

Nearly all the problems that arise in Alzheimer's have their roots in disruption to parts of the brain, including those already mentioned in the sections, 'Communication' and 'Memory and Emotions'. Over time the disease spreads and affects an increasing number of areas. The specific areas impacted and the timescale of this varies slightly from person to person so are not entirely predictable. But sooner of later all the common symptoms will manifest. The following aberrant behaviours and thought patterns are common in people with Alzheimer's; I have given some suggestions for responding to them.

Repetition

Repetition is a common trait in people with Alzheimer's, caused by damage in the frontal lobe. It can take the form of saying the same thing over and over again or performing repetitive movements, and being with someone who is doing this sort of thing can test the patience of a saint. It is as if the brain gets stuck in a groove but the person doesn't realize this so can't correct it. Extreme patience is required on our part.

Fixating

As brain activity slows down, people with Alzheimer's fixate on whatever they happen to be looking at, and the length of time they spend fixating gets longer as the disease progresses. However, rather than us trying to speed things up, we can slow down and enjoy spending time looking at things with them. If you are talking to someone with late-stage Alzheimer's, it is likely that they will fixate on your eyes or mouth and maybe comment on them.

Being Oblivious to Errors

People who have Alzheimer's often say and do things that are bizarre and irrational, but they are completely unaware of this

241

– they do not hear themselves not making sense or realize that what they are doing is not normal. It is not helpful, therefore, to point out their errors or contradict them as this just leads to further distress. Again, this requires patience.

Misperception of Time

As the disease progresses people with Alzheimer's lose their sense of linear time and often don't differentiate between past, present and future – all time gets rolled into the present. This can be confusing to us but if we are aware of it we may find clues to the timeframe they are thinking about in the content of what they are saying. So listen for the clues and ask questions, gently.

Misperception of Age and Capabilities

From time to time people with Alzheimer's experience being as they were rather than as they are now. This leads to totally unrealistic expectations of what they can do and needs to be handled safely and gently. However, it can have its advantages. If the person is enjoying a period in their lives when they were fit and youthful, talking about it can give them some relief from their current disabilities and limitations. It could also be an opportunity to engage with them in their timeframe in a meaningful way.

Intermittent Disruption

Disruption to brain function in people with Alzheimer's is often intermittent. This means one day they might be well and quite lucid, another day flaccid and less coherent, then another day quite lucid again. Things don't progress in a straight line.

One common reason for 'down' periods is infection. It is well known that brain function can be severely affected by infections such as urinary tract infections (UTIs), which are very common in people with Alzheimer's in the later stages. So it is important to keep an open mind and check how the person is feeling, knowing that things can change in both directions.

Varying Capabilities

As disruption to the brain is intermittent, people with Alzheimer's have times when they can do things and other times when they can't. It is important to be aware of this and not presume that they are incapable all the time. So give them the opportunity to do things and check their capability sensitively without putting them under any strain.

Responding to Altered States of Consciousness

People with Alzheimer's, particularly in the later stages, from time to time experience what I would call altered states of consciousness. These can range from being extremely lucid on the one hand to drifting into a world that is completely unfamiliar to us on the other. It is important that we recognize these different states and understand them so that we can manage our expectations and respond appropriately.

Lucidity

When people are not functioning well and can hardly speak, it is very surprising when suddenly, out of the blue, they demonstrate lucidity: they perceive the truth and see everything with great clarity. Naturally, when this happens we are filled with hope that things have improved. However, this is a temporary altered state of consciousness that has been found to happen more frequently near the end of life, and not only in people with Alzheimer's.[27]

When people are in this profound state, we should pay attention to what they are telling us, and validate them.

Other Worlds

People with late-stage Alzheimer's sometimes seem to drift into another dimension of consciousness. If they have lost most of their faculty of speech, and the little they are saying doesn't make sense to us, it is easy for us to dismiss them. However, my mother was able to speak and she told me about extremely positive experiences she had in the Other World: her lack of constraints and worries, her great freedom of thought, and her feelings of utter peace and universal love.

How should we respond to people when they seem to be experiencing this Other World? The Other World is real to them so we should validate their experiences, even if they are not real to us. If we do we might be surprised by what they tell us. We might learn from them.

Other Core Care Provision

There are many things we can do to improve quality of life for people with Alzheimer's, whether they are being looked after in their own home or in a residential care home. These include offering them creative activities, outings, exercise, proper hydration, natural remedies and visualization (see page 248).

Creative Activities

People with Alzheimer's benefit greatly from all kinds of creative activities: singing, music, poetry, dance, art, making things, gardening, cooking, etc. There are a number of reasons for this. The filters that come between thoughts and perceptions and the external world are no longer working in them, so their experience of external stimuli is more direct. Their emotional feelings live on and they can remember things from the past that had emotional meaning for them. For example, they are particularly good at remembering tunes and the words of songs.[28] Because their brain activity has slowed down they take time to appreciate the beauty of nature and are touched by it. My mother continued to love dance and movement and got great pleasure from this, even when she couldn't physically engage in it. She surprised herself, and us, when she discovered that she could read poetry with meaning, even when she couldn't remember what she had just said in normal conversations. Tailoring the kind of stimulation to the person's individual interests will greatly improve their quality of life, and family and friends can contribute in this area in particular.

John Killick, a poet and researcher into the language of people with dementia, has found that the arts, particularly language, offer a very direct and meaningful way for people with dementia to communicate.[29] Another researcher, John Zeisel, author of *I'm Still Here* and an innovator in the non-pharmacological treatment of Alzheimer's, has shown that feelings of wellbeing can be enhanced in people with Alzheimer's by providing them with carefully planned environments and creative activities.[30]

Outings

It is very beneficial to take people with Alzheimer's out to places they know and love. Going out breaks the monotony of being at home or in the care home and provides much needed stimulation from the outside world. But outings need advance planning; it takes time and effort to get the person ready and out the door. The outing also needs to be tailored to the person's capabilities so that they and you are safe. Bear in mind that for residents of a care home any outing must be authorized by the person in charge before you leave.

Exercise

Any exercise that activates the brain and the body is helpful to people with Alzheimer's and care homes usually employ specially trained activities co-ordinators to run regular group exercise sessions for residents. These are designed so that they can be performed sitting for those who are immobile.

Hydration

It is common for people with Alzheimer's to become dehydrated and this is problematic because it causes the brain and the body to function less well. In the later stages of Alzheimer's, when people are unable to drink unassisted, help is required and providing this is very time-consuming for care assistants. Also, it is hard to keep an accurate record of fluid intake, so people can easily slip through the net.

Always take the opportunity to offer an elderly person something to drink, preferably water, and check regularly that their fluid intake is sufficient, especially if they can't ask for a drink themselves or manage to drink without assistance.

Medical Treatment and Natural Remedies

As yet there is no effective medical treatment or cure for Alzheimer's, but some natural remedies have been found to help slow down some of the symptoms in some people. For example, research undertaken at Newcastle University in 2003 showed that lemon balm (*melissa officinalis*) and sage (*salvia officinalis*) both improve memory. As always, professional advice should be sought before embarking on any treatment programme. Maintaining a healthy lifestyle as far as possible remains the best course of action.

Caring for Yourself

And what about you? Who is caring for you? If you are a professional carer you may be working long hours doing really demanding work and getting little financial reward or acknowledgement. If you are a family member the demands on you may be like a bottomless pit. Whoever you are, it is very important that you step out of the caring role from time to time, take stock and acknowledge what *you* need – you, too, need to find a positive way forward. So be kind to yourself and take time for yourself. You are a *very* important person – maybe even an angel!

Keeping a Record

I strongly recommend you keep a journal of some kind in which you write down the things your loved one says and does, and add photos and other mementos. You might want to record the person's voice or the sound of you singing together. Do whatever has meaning for you. It will provide you with lasting memories and be something to treasure in the future.

Conclusion

It is our emotions, our feelings, that give meaning to our lives and this is no different for people with Alzheimer's. Although their physical body and parts of their brain are deteriorating, their emotions live on. This means people with Alzheimer's can stay connected to others and to the world through feelings, right to the end of their lives.

We can help them to do this in a number of ways: by ensuring that they are well cared for and feel safe; by being fully present and loving with them; by being emotionally engaged with them; by providing opportunities for creative expression through which they can express their emotions.

These things enhance not only their lives but also ours. So this chapter is not only about a positive way forward for people with Alzheimer's, but also about a positive way forward for us. But in order for us to move forward *we* probably need to change. We need to become more present, more emotionally honest and more direct in our communication with others. In truth, we need to be more like our loved ones.

Guided Visualization

Visualization can be very helpful for people with Alzheimer's, as they can gain pleasure and relief from this when they can no longer do things physically. However, some people take to visualization more readily than others, so at first experiment for just a minute or two. The experience should not only be enjoyable for the person being guided, but also relaxing for you, too. So enjoy!

A visualization exercise has three stages:
- The setting-up stage
- The guided visualization
- The setting-down stage

The Setting-up Stage

- Before you start, establish a safe, comfortable base for the person; for example, they could be sitting in a chair or lying in bed, with you by their side.
- Tell them they can return to this base at any time and should indicate to you if they wish to do so.

The Guided Visualization

- Start with the general 'Feeling Good' visualization (see opposite).

- Pay attention to your voice – it should be slow, gentle, soothing in tone.
- Allow plenty of time for the person to process your instructions.
- Observe the person throughout and stay tuned in to them.
- If you have any concerns, check in with the person and follow their wishes to continue or to stop.
- When you have finished the 'Feeling Good' visualization, you can proceed to a specific visualization, such as the example given here ('Moving', see page 251), or go straight to the setting-down stage.
- Bear in mind that these visualization exercises can be beneficially repeated many times.

The Setting-down Stage

- Say the words of 'Returning to the Present' (see page 250), adjusting your tone of voice to a more matter-of-fact one and increasing your speed of talking a little.
- When you have finished speaking, check that the person is fully back in their body, eyes open and aware.
- Give them a few moments to adjust before moving on to something else.

Feeling Good Visualization

Say the following words in a slow, gentle, soothing tone of voice:

'Close your eyes, pause, relax and let your mind be quiet.
Feel your body anchored to whatever you are resting on.
Be aware of your environment: sounds, temperature and
    anything else.
When you are ready,
Move your attention to your breathing.

Let your breathing slow down. Taking your time ...
As you breathe out let your breath flow down through your
    body, legs and feet.
Feel your head, neck and all down your spine relaxing.
Feel your whole body relaxing.
Now start imagining you are in your perfect situation – it
    can be real or fantasy.
Begin exploring and experiencing it fully.
What are you are seeing?
What are you hearing?
What are you feeling?
Is there any taste, any smell?
Is this perfect, just how you want it? If not, change it and
    make it how you want it.
Is there anything else you would like to include that would
    make it even better?
Be aware of what you are feeling.
Enjoy this state.
Know that you can return to it again.'

Now end the session with 'Returning to the Present' or go on to
another visualization, such as the 'Moving Visualization'.

Returning to the Present

Say the following words more quickly, in a more matter-of-fact
tone of voice:

'When you are ready, bring your attention back to where
    you are now.
Bring your awareness into your body and feel the weight of
    your body on whatever you are resting on.
Now wiggle your fingers and toes.
When you are ready, open your eyes.
Look around and take a few moments to become fully aware
    of where you are and how you are feeling.'

Moving Visualization

Say the following words in a slow, gentle, soothing tone of voice:

'Move your attention to your breathing.
Let your breathing slow down. Taking your time ...
As you breathe out let your breath flow down through your
   body, legs and feet.
When you are ready,
Imagine you are getting into a position for moving your body.
Imagine stretching as fully as is comfortable.
Now, taking your attention to your toes and feet, imagine
   starting to move them, very slowly at first.
Now your ankles.
And now your legs.
Can you feel the freedom of this movement?
Now your spine – feel it moving slightly.
And now your neck – feel it moving, too.
Taking your attention now to your fingers, imagine starting
   to move them just a little at first.
Now imagine moving your hands and your wrists.
And now your arms.
Can you feel the freedom of this movement?
Now your shoulders a little, very gently.
You may want to imagine moving your head.
As everything eases and is feeling free, imagine moving
   every part of you.
Imagine moving freely.
Enjoying this feeling.
Taking your time ... and as long as you want ...
Know that you can experience this again.'

End the session with 'Returning to the Present' (see page 250).

251

CLOSING THOUGHTS

'Love never dies.'
Pat

In this final part of the book I have reflected on the journey that took my mother and me into two worlds, this world and the Other World, and appreciated the gifts we discovered in both those dimensions. I have marvelled at the miraculous healings that have taken place within our family. I have also presented the information I gathered – and revelations I had – during the quest for knowledge that I embarked on following the ending of our Heart and Soul Journey. Pulling together everything I have learned, I have proposed a positive way forward for people who have Alzheimer's and for those who care for them.

What, then, are my closing thoughts?

Death and Dying

Despite, or maybe because of, the depressing prospect of three impending deaths in my family, I made a conscious choice to prepare myself and face the dark and difficult time that I knew lay ahead. I am so glad I did. Instead of experiencing only sorrow and loss as I had expected, to my amazement I found love and light that has filled my heart and soul. This experience has changed my life.

The majority of people in the Western world have become divorced from the process of dying, death and grieving, and I believe it is time to turn the spotlight on this taboo subject. Disengagement often stems from fear; and fear, from ignorance. I hope my family's story will reassure others, bring comfort, and dispel the fear that is so often associated with death and which distances people from death and from their loved ones.

252

Birth and death are the opposite sides of the same coin and equally important. When a baby comes into the world, we know that for the first few years it should be given total care; a baby is loved, nurtured and all its physical and emotional needs are met. So why don't we give this same level of care and nurturing at the end of life? The needs are no different. This is a precious time when we can connect with our loved ones in a very special way and help them prepare for and go on to experience a good death.

Apart from cases of accident, suicide and sudden death, dying is a process, and in the case of Alzheimer's a long process. When undertaken with conscious awareness it can, as the Heart and Soul Journey shows, be a truly wonderful and enriching experience. An exploration of death, consciousness and the Other World provides us with the greatest opportunity to learn about our lives and our souls, right here and right now.

The Gifts of Alzheimer's

People with late-stage Alzheimer's who are egoless and totally present can access altered states of consciousness and transcendental states. In this Other World they leave all their bodily and emotional limitations behind and experience pure love and total bliss. In addition, they can bring wisdom and love from the Other World to us, and we can engage with them in a symbiotic healing process in which everyone benefits. These are the gifts of Alzheimer's.

Our Family

As our Heart and Soul Journey unfolded, mysteriously all the stars in our family constellation were reconfigured with perfect synchronicity, demonstrating the interconnectedness of all things. Our experience shows that it is never too late to try to put things right. It whispers in my soul that there really is a higher level of consciousness operating beyond this world.

Our World Now

Over the last few decades the world in which we live has changed dramatically from being predominantly analogue to digital. Ever faster digital processing is affecting how our brains work, how we think and how we feel. It is robbing us of our precious ability to be still, to observe, to draw on our natural creativity, to see the big picture and to expand our consciousness. The kinds of timeless experiences associated with late-stage Alzheimer's provide us with a way back into the world that our soul, at the deepest level, is yearning for. These are the gifts people with Alzheimer's have. These were the gifts my mother gave me.

Wonder

In order to illuminate what happened on our journey, I have at times been analytical and travelled in linear time. But returning to the essence of the story, I am filled with a feeling of wonder. This is what the Heart and Soul Journey is really about.

One World

I am aware that throughout this book I have talked about the two worlds as if they are separate, when of course they are not. We experience the physical world through our five outer senses and the Other World through our inner senses – both worlds are part of us. Love embraces both worlds and unites them. So, if we are present in the moment, keep an open mind and connect with love in our heart, we can have the best of both worlds, this and the Other World, and experience the bliss of One World.

Love

'Love is what it is,' my mother said. Love brings joy and other good feelings and we can make it a part of our daily lives by expressing it in whatever we are doing: by caring for people and things, by preparing food, by making something, by being creative, by sending a blessing, by giving someone a smile. As the saying goes: 'It's not what you do, it's the way that you do it.' By feeling love ourselves, we can enable everyone around us to feel it, too.

Our story started with love and ended with love, and I am now passing on this message of LOVE to you!

EPILOGUE

Reflecting on my mother's life, it seems to me as though nothing has been lost; it has merely changed. As a snowflake melts to form water and water evaporates into the air, so her life has gone through transformations but her essence remains.

Although the stage of the journey that my mother and I took together in this world is now complete, the journey itself is by no means ended. When I see 'little bits floating, flying off', I know it is Mum. She is still with me, still teaching me, still loving me ...

'Love never dies.'
Mum

NOTES

1 Evans-Roberts, CEY and Turnbull, OH (2011) *Remembering relationships: preserved emotion-based learning in Alzheimer's disease.* Available: www.tandfonline.com.

2 Sturm, VE et al (2013) *Heightened emotional contagion in mild cognitive impairment and Alzheimer's disease is associated with temporal lobe degeneration.* Available: http://www.pnas.org.

3 Zeisel, J (2011) *I'm Still Here*, Piatkus.

4 Pert, C (1997) *Molecules of Emotion*, Simon & Schuster.

5 Brennan, B (1987) *Hands of Light*, Bantam Books.

6 Sanders, C (1975) *The Care of the Dying Patient and His Family*, The London Medical Group.

7 Fenwick, P and Fenwick, E (2008) *The Art of Dying*, Continuum.

8 Moody, R (1973) *Life After Life*, Bantam Books.

9 Sheldrake R (2003) *The Sense of Being Stared At, and Other Aspects of the Extended Mind*, Arrow Books.

10 Moody, RA (1975) *Life After Life*, Mockingbird Books.

11 *Oxford Dictionaries*, http://www.oxforddictionaries.com.

12 McTaggart, L (2001) *The Field*, HarperCollins.

13 László, E (2004) *Science and the Akashic Field*, Inner Traditions.

14 Tolle, E (1999) *The Power of Now*, New World Library.

15 Lodge, O (1933) 'The Mode of Future Existence', *The Queen's Hospital Annual*.

16 Greene, B (2011) *The Hidden Reality*, Penguin.

17 Marina-Tompkins, V (2000) *The Seven Transitional Stages During the Astral Interval.* Available: www.flightofthehawk.com.

18 Blavatsky, HP *The Theosophist*, June 1880.

19 New York University's Aging and Dementia Research Center.

20 O'Connor, J and McDermott, I (2013) *Principles of NLP*, Singing Dragon.

21 Rogers, C (1996) *Way of Being*, Houghton Mifflin.

22 Feil, N (2002) *The Validation Breakthrough*, Health Professions Press.

23 Sanders, C (1975) *The Care of the Dying Patient and His Family*, The London Medical Group.

24 Uvnäs Moberg, Dr K (2003) *The Oxytocin Factor*, Da Capo Press.

25 Killick, J and Allan, K (2001) *Communication and the Care of People with Dementia*, Open University Press.

26 Brennan, B (1987) *Hands of Light*, Bantam Books.

27 Fenwick, P and Fenwick, E (2008) *The Art of Dying*, Continuum.

28 See www.alzheimers.org.uk for information about Singing for the Brain.

29 Killick, J (2011) *Creativity and Communication in Persons with Dementia*, Jessica Kingsley.

30 Zeisel, J (2011) *I'm Still Here*, Piatkus.

GLOSSARY

Note: Many of the terms listed here are esoteric and there is no absolute definition of them – they are open to interpretation.

Akashic Records or Book of Life or The Library: Metaphor for all the information in the universe – every experience, thought and event since the beginning of time. This archive or memory bank is said to exist on a non-physical plane called the Akashic Field, which is the Universal Field of Consciousness. Psychics who claim to have accessed these records inform us that The Library is being continually updated. According to many spiritual teachers, the study of these books is an essential and natural stage after death.

angel: High-frequency energy form that is sensed or appears in non-physical form. Also sometimes referred to as a 'helper'.

astral projection or astral travel: Involves a part of the self leaving the physical body temporarily and travelling in the astral plane (a non-physical dimension), then returning and reconnecting to the physical body. We experience astral projection naturally in our dreams but it is also something people can do while fully conscious, although it is most often reported as occurring involuntarily near the end of life.

aura: Energy field that surrounds all living and non-living things. In humans it can extend out to a metre from the body. It holds old and current physical, emotional, mental and spiritual information about the person. The aura is not detected by people generally but healers and psychics are sensitive to it. Clairvoyants describe seeing the aura as dynamic moving energy that has a range of colours.

chakra system: Important subtle-energy system comprising a number of chakras or 'force centres' located in the physical body, mainly in the spine. These chakras produce invisible energy that permeates the body and the layers of the aura or human energy field (HEF). The energy moves in vortices in an ever-increasing fan-shaped formation. Chakras are considered to be the focal points for the transmission and reception of energies. There are seven major chakras and a number of minor ones and each has a particular function. An imbalance in any one will impact the person in some way. Most healers work on balancing the energy in the chakras to create a greater sense of health, wellbeing and harmony.

channel: In the world of extrasensory perception (ESP), someone who is in contact with the *other side*. Unlike a medium, whose connection is of a personal nature, a channel is open to wisdom from the highest source. Channels convey universal messages that are intended for the benefit of all and the planet.

chi (qi): Energy that runs through the meridians of the acupuncture system. This energy is inside the body and extends outside the body. It is therefore the bridge between the physical body and the subtle energy fields.

clairsentience: Clear knowing or clear thinking. Associated with the power of prophecy, it comes from a non-physical dimension and is one aspect of ESP.

clairvoyance: Ability to see clearly when out of the normal range of vision. This visual information is accessed through the brow chakra, the third eye. It comes from a non-physical dimension and is one aspect of ESP.

Dass, Ram: Contemporary American spiritual teacher and author of the seminal book *Be Here Now*.

dissociation: When normal consciousness or psychological functioning is disrupted. This altered state of consciousness results in the person being 'cut off' from what is happening.

entity: Soul, mind and body (physical or otherwise), in its active, spiritual form.

extrasensory perception (ESP): Reception of information obtained through a non-physical sense; sometimes called the sixth sense or intuition.

healing: Natural process by which the body (or mind or spirit) heals itself; can involve self-healing or healing applied by another, often a healer or therapist. The healing arts aim to stimulate the healing process to bring the whole system into a state of greater balance and harmony. Healers do this by becoming present, tuning in to the person, connecting with the Source, then feeling that energy radiate through them.

inner senses: Means through which we experience our inner world and the Other World. They are not defined by time or space. Transcendental states, spiritual experiences, dream states, out-of-body experiences, astral projection and all kinds of ESP come through our inner senses.

medium: Person in contact with the deceased on the *other side*. Acts as a channel for information to pass from spirits in the Other World to interested parties in this world, and often also puts questions to the spirits. The messages the medium receives can come through in a number of different forms: thoughts, words, symbols, visions, automatic writing, feelings, sensations and even scents. Sometimes the medium goes into a trance and takes on the voice, posture and other characteristics of the deceased person whose spirit is speaking.

mindfulness: Mode of perception that involves pausing and being aware in the present moment without judgement or evaluation; originates in Eastern spiritual and religious traditions.

monkey mind: The chattering brain; a term coined over 2000 years ago in China. It is used to dispel the anxiety and fear that arises from ambiguity and not knowing.

near-death experience (NDE): This occurs when someone is declared clinically dead, often due to cardiac arrest, but recovers and can later describe what they saw and heard during the time they were clinically dead. The person's viewpoint is often from a position above their body. Research into this phenomenon has substantiated these claims. An NDE frequently changes the person: they no longer fear death and they become less materialistic and more spiritual. The term 'transitory death experience' (TDE) has been introduced more recently as a more accurate description of the situation.

numerology: Study of numbers and the occult way in which they reflect certain aptitudes and character tendencies, as an integral part of the cosmic plan. In this system each letter has a numeric value that provides a related cosmic vibration.

orbs: Tiny specks of light that appear seemingly out of nowhere and disappear again as quickly as they appeared. It is said that this is the energy of which all things are made.

Other World: Although there is no definitive description of this, a number of terms can be used to explain this idea: other reality, other dimension, other realm, 'other side', 'Spirit'.

out-of-body experience: Sensation of floating outside one's body and perceiving it from a place above or outside it. Everyone who has had an NDE has reported floating above his or her body, so it would seem that this sensation is part of the natural dying experience, but it can occur in the normal course of life, too.

past-life regression: Therapeutic approach in which the practitioner, using hypnosis, induces a state of deep trance in the patient or client. This is to enable them to recover information from past lives or incarnations, usually to resolve some problem in this life. The work has a spiritual basis and implies a belief in reincarnation.

***The Prophet*:** Collection of twenty-six poetic essays written by Kahlil Gibran, a Lebanese artist, philosopher and writer. First published in 1926 and still widely read today, it offers profound discussions about life and the human condition. The words of the Prophet Almustafa are as insightful and relevant today as they were when the book was first written.

psychic: Person with extrasensory perception (ESP). The information received can come through a number of different sensory channels, such as clairvoyance, clairaudience or clairsentience, or through telepathy or precognition.

reincarnation: Believed to occur when the soul or spirit, after the death of the body, comes back to life in a newborn body. If this is so, then we have many lives and the previous ones are referred to as 'past lives'. According to this belief, before incarnating and while still in the inter-life, we choose a new life situation that will give us the opportunity to learn lessons we have not learned in a previous life. This is where the notion of karma comes from.

soul: The Spirit or God part of the individual; all the entity has been or may be; the real continuous self. Coming from Spirit, the soul is both universal and individual. It is the spiritual essence of an entity manifest in the material plane. Man *is* soul

– he doesn't acquire a soul. On the material plane, man seeks soul manifestation.

spheres, the music of the ancient: Philosophical concept that regards proportions in the movements of celestial bodies – the sun, moon and planets – as a form of music. This music is not audible but a mathematical concept. Legend has it that Pythagoras heard the music of the spheres and this led to his mathematical discoveries.

Spirit: Pure consciousness. God is Spirit and man comes from Spirit. Spirit is the life of the soul. Man is soul – an individual expression of Spirit.

FURTHER READING

Recommended reading

This reading list provides information that will add to your understanding of the Heart and Soul Journey.

Alexander, Dr Eben, *Proof of Heaven*, Piatkus: London, 2012

Bloom, Dr William, *The Power of Modern Spirituality*, Piatkus: London, 2011

Bolte Taylor, Jill, *My Stroke of Insight*, Hodder & Stoughton, London, 2008

Brayne, Sue and Fenwick, Dr Peter, *End-of-Life Experiences: A Guide for Carers of the Dying*, University of Southampton ebook: Southampton, UK, 2008

Brayne, Sue and Fenwick, Dr Peter, *Nearing the End of Life: A Guide for Relatives and Friends of the Dying*, University of Southampton ebook: Southampton, UK, 2013

Brennan, Barbara Ann, *Hands of Light*, Bantam: New York, 1990

Chopra, Deepak, *Life After Death*, Rider: London, 2008

Davis, Dr Brenda, *Journey of the Soul*, Hodder Paperbacks: London, 2003

Eden, Donna, *Energy Medicine*, Piatkus: London, 2008

Feil, Naomi, *The Validation Breakthrough*, Health Professions Press: Baltimore (MD), USA, 2002

Fenwick, Dr Peter and Fenwick, Elizabeth, *The Art of Dying*, Continuum: London, 2008

Greene, Brian, *The Hidden Reality*, Penguin: London, 2012

Hamilton, Dr David R, *It's The Thought That Counts*, Hay House UK: London, 2008

Holford, Patrick, *The Alzheimer's Prevention Plan*, Piatkus: London, 2005

Killick, John, *Creativity and Communication in Persons with Dementia*, Jessica Kingsley: London, 2011

Killick, John and Allan, Kate, *Communication and the Care of People with Dementia*, Open University Press: Milton Keynes, 2001

Kubler-Ross, Elizabeth, *On Death and Dying* (reprint), Scribner: New York, 2014

Lipinska, Danuta, *Person-centred Counselling for People with Dementia*, Jessica Kingsley: London, 2009

McTaggart, Lynne, *The Field*, Element: Shaftesbury, Dorset 2003

McTaggart, Lynne, *The Bond*, Hay House UK: London, 2013

Moody, Raymond, *Life After Life*, Rider: London, 2001

Moorjani, Anita, *Dying to Be Me*, Hay House UK: London, 2012

Pert, Candace B, *Molecules of Emotion*, Pocket Books: New York, 1999

Razzaque, Dr Russell, *Breaking Down Is Waking Up*, Watkins: London, 2014

Rinpoche, Sogyal, *The Tibetan Book of Living and Dying*, Rider: London, 2008

Rix, Brigitte, *I'm Not Dead: I'm Alive Without a Body*, Con-Psy Publications: Greenford, Middlesex, 2011

Satori, Dr Penny, *The Wisdom of Near-Death Experiences*, Watkins: London, 2014

Schwartz, Dr Gary E, *The Afterlife Experiments*, Simon & Schuster: New York, 2003

Schwartz, Robert, *Your Soul's Gift*, Whispering Winds Press: Chesterland (OH), USA, 2012

Sheard, Dr David, *Feelings Matter Most* (series), Dementia Care Matters Books: Brighton, 2011–2012

Sheldrake, Rupert, *Dogs That Know When Their Owners Are Coming Home*, Arrow: London, 2000

Simard, Joyce, *The End-of-Life Namaste Care Program for People with Dementia*, Health Professions Press: Baltimore (MD), USA, 2013

Tolle, Eckhart, *The Power of Now*, Hodder Paperbacks: London, 2011

Walsch, Neale Donald, *Conversations with God* (series), *Book 1*, Hodder & Stoughton: London, 1997

Walsch, Neale Donald, *Home with God*, Hodder Paperbacks: London, 2007

Warner, Felicity, *The Soul Midwives' Handbook*, Hay House UK: London, 2013

Williams, Mark and Penman, Danny, *Mindfulness*, Piatkus: London, 2011

Zeisel, John, *I'm Still Here*, Piatkus: London, 2011

Supplementary Reading

This reading list provides additional information that will facilitate your understanding of the wider aspects of the story.

Bays, Brandon, *The Journey*, Atria Books: New York, 2012

Berg, Yehuda, *The Power of Kabbalah*, Hodder Paperbacks: London, 2004

Bohm, David, *Wholeness and the Implicate Order*, Routledge: London, 2002

Bowlby, John, *Attachment and Loss (Volume 1)*, Pimlico: London, 1997

Brayne, Sue, *The D-Word*, Continuum: London, 2010

Capra, Fritjof, *The Tao of Physics*, Flamingo: London, 1992

Carper, Jean, *100 Simple Things You Can Do To Prevent Alzheimer's*, Vermilion: London, 2011

Chetwynd, Tom, *A Dictionary of Symbols*, Paladin: London, 1982

Childre, Doc and Martin, Howard, *The HeartMath Solution*, HarperOne: San Francisco, 2000

Currivan, Jude and László, Ervin, *Cosmos: A Co-Creator's Guide to the Whole World*, Hay House UK: London, 2008

Dass, Ram, *Be Here Now*, HarperCollins ebooks, London, 2010

Dilts, Robert, Hallbom, Tim and Smith, Suzi, *Beliefs*, Crown House: Carmarthen, 2012

Dossey, Dr Larry, *Healing Beyond the Body*, Piatkus: London, 2009

Dossey, Dr Larry, *One Mind*, Hay House UK: London, 2013

Dyer, Dr Wayne, *The Power of Intention*, Hay House UK: London, 2010

Edwards, Gill, *Living Magically*, Piatkus: London, 2009

Emoto, Masaru, *The Hidden Messages in Water*, Pocket Books: New York, 2005

Foundation for Inner Peace, *A Course in Miracles*, The Foundation for Inner Peace: Mill Valley (CA), USA, 2008

Gawain, Shakti, *Creative Visualization*, New World Library: Novato (CA), USA, 2002

Gerber, Richard, *Vibrational Medicine*, Bear & Company: Rochester (VT), USA, 2001

Gibran, Kahlil, *The Prophet*, Pan: London, 1991

Gray, John, *Men are from Mars, Women are from Venus*, Harper Element: London, 2012

Hamilton, Dr David, *How Your Mind Can Heal Your Body*, Hay House UK: London, 2008

Hay, Louise, *You Can Heal Your Life*, Hay House UK: London, 2004

Hicks, Esther and Hicks, Jerry, *Ask and It Is Given*, Hay House UK: London, 2008

Holford, Patrick and Burne, Jerome, *The 10 Secrets of Healthy Ageing*, Piatkus: London, 2012

James, Oliver, *Contented Dementia*, Vermilion: London, 2009

Jung, Carl G, *Man and His Symbols*, Picador: London, 1978

Jung, Carl G, *Memories, Dreams, Reflections*, Flamingo: London, 1995

Kabat-Zinn, Jon, *Full Catastrophe Living*, Piatkus: London, 2013

Katie, Byron, *Loving What Is*, Rider: London, 2002

King, Serge Kahili, *Kahuna Healing*, Quest: Wheaton (IL), USA, 1983

László, Ervin, *Science and the Akashic Field*, Inner Traditions: Rochester (VT), USA, 2007

La Tourelle, Maggie, *Principles of Kinesiology*, Singing Dragon: London, 2013

Leininger, Bruce and Leininger, Andrea, *Soul Survivor*, Hay House UK: London, 2010

Levine, Stephen, *Healing into Life and Death*, Random House: London, 1989

Levine, Stephen, *Who Dies?* Anchor Books: New York, 1982

Linn, Denise, *Pocketful of Dreams*, Piatkus: London, 1993

Lipton, Dr Bruce, *The Biology of Belief*, Hay House UK: London, 2011

McGilchrist, Iain, *The Master and His Emissary*, Yale University Press: New Haven (CT), USA, 2012

Miller, Alice, *The Drama of Being a Child*, Virago: London, 2008

O'Connor, Joseph and McDermott, Ian, *Principles of NLP*, Singing Dragon: London, 2013

Peck, M Scott, *The Road Less Travelled*, Rider: London, 2008

Robbins, Tony, *Awakening the Giant Within*, Pocket Books, New York, 2001

Roberts, Jane, *The Seth Material*, New Awareness Network Inc.: Manhasset (NY), USA, 2001

Sheldrake, Rupert, *The Presence of the Past*, Park Street Press: New York, 2012

Skynner, Robin and Cleese, John, *Families and How to Survive Them*, Cedar Books: New Delhi, India, 1993

Smith, Huston, *The World's Religions*, HarperOne: San Francisco, 2009

Talbot, Marianne, *Keeping Mum*, Hay House UK: London, 2011

Thurman, Robert (translator), *The Tibetan Book of the Dead*, Penguin: London, 2006

Woolger, Dr Roger J, *Other Lives, Other Selves*, Bantam: London, 1988

Wooten-Green, Ron *When the Dying Speak*, Loyola Press: Chicago, 2003

DVD

Will Arntz, Betsy Chasse and Mark Vicente, *What the Bleep Do We Know!?*, Lord of the Wind Films, 2004

RESOURCES

UK

Age Concern: www.ageuk.org.uk

The Alzheimer's Society UK: www.alzheimers.org.uk; includes
information about Singing for the Brain

The Association for Therapeutic Healers: www.healers-ath.org

Care Quality Commission: www.cqc.org.uk

Citizens Advice Bureau: www.adviceguide.org.uk

The Confederation of Healing Organizations:
www.the-cho.org.uk

Dementia Care Matters: www.dementiacarematters.com

Dementia Challengers: www.dementiachallengers.com

Dementia UK: www.dementiauk.org

Felicity Warner, Soul Midwives: www.soulmidwives.co.uk

Hermione Elliott, Living Well Dying Well:
www.livingwelldyingwell.net

Innovations in Dementia CIC:
www.innovationsindementia.org.uk

The National Council for Palliative Care:
www.dyingmatters.org

William Bloom Courses on Dying (Passing Over) and becoming
a Spiritual Companion: www.williambloom.com

Bereavement support

The British Association for Counselling and Psychotherapy:
www.bacp.co.uk

Cruse: www.crusebereavementcare.org.uk

Samaritans: www.samaritans.org

INTERNATIONAL

Alzheimer's Association: www.alz.org
Being with Dying: www.upaya.org/bwd
HeartMath: www.heartmath.com
Namaste Care Program For People With Dementia:
    www.namastecare.com

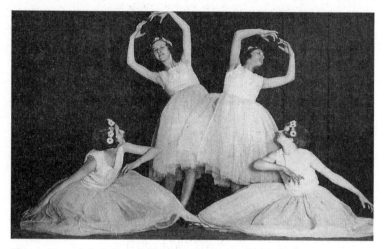

Mum (top right) during an amateur performance in Ayrshire, *c.* 1938

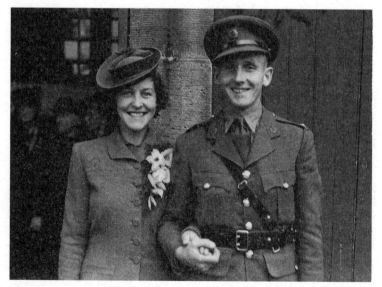

Pat (Mum) and William (Dad) on their wedding day, 1941

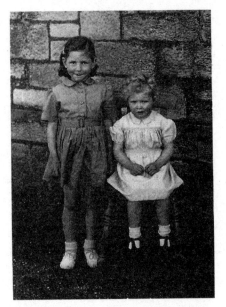

Margaret and her sister, 1949

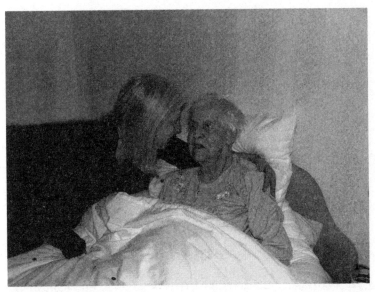

Margaret and Mum, 2006

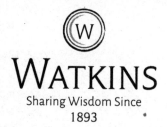

WATKINS

Sharing Wisdom Since
1893

The story of Watkins Publishing dates back to March 1893, when John M. Watkins, a scholar of esotericism, overheard his friend and teacher Madame Blavatsky lamenting the fact that there was nowhere in London to buy books on mysticism, occultism or metaphysics. At that moment Watkins was born, soon to become the home of many of the leading lights of spiritual literature, including Carl Jung, Rudolf Steiner, Alice Bailey and Chögyam Trungpa.

Today our passion for vigorous questioning is still resolute. With over 350 titles on our list, Watkins Publishing reflects the development of spiritual thinking and new science over the past 120 years. We remain at the cutting edge, committed to publishing books that change lives.

DISCOVER MORE ...

Read our blog

Watch and listen to
our authors in action

Sign up to
our mailing list

JOIN IN THE CONVERSATION

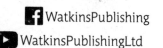 WatkinsPublishing   @watkinswisdom

▶ WatkinsPublishingLtd   8+ +watkinspublishing1893

Our books celebrate conscious, passionate, wise and happy living.
Be part of the community by visiting

www.watkinspublishing.com